FOOT PAIN

Also by Dr. Mennell

BACK PAIN
Diagnosis and Treatment
Using Manipulative Techniques

JOINT PAIN
Diagnosis and Treatment
Using Manipulative Techniques

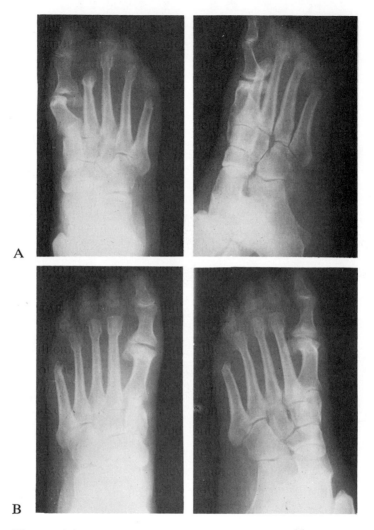

X-rays of the feet (A, the right foot; B, the left foot) of a 42-year-old woman who, at the age of 18, had normal, painless feet. Four years later she had painful bunions. The pictures illustrate well the long-term results of "corrective" but in reality destructive surgery which has only led to more pain and disability. See page 5.

FOOT PAIN

John McM. Mennell, M.D.

Associate Professor, Physical Medicine and
Rehabilitation, The University of Pennsylvania
School of Medicine, Philadelphia; Chief of
Physical Medicine and Rehabilitation Service,
Brentwood Veterans Administration Hospital,
Los Angeles

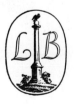

LITTLE, BROWN AND COMPANY

Boston

Preface

I venture to say that few adults in the shoe-wearing population of the world do not suffer from foot discomfort, ranging from tired feet through aching feet to frankly painful feet. In teaching and demonstrating examining procedures as they relate to the feet, I always insist that my students use only one foot of their partners, and invariably each member of the class asks that the other foot be put through the same examining maneuvers at the end of the session because the foot which has been used is so comfortable, light, and resilient. Yet it is seldom that any one of them admits to symptoms of foot pain before class begins.

There are only about eight thousand certified podiatrists in the United States to care for a foot population of about four hundred million, and few physicians and surgeons have any training in the problems of the feet. Orthopedists have devised a myriad of operations hopefully designed to "cure" frank foot pain, but most of these procedures are based on anatomical concepts derived from dead feet or, worse, the bare skeleton of dead feet, according to the unchanging teaching of past decades.

The public is at the mercy of shoe manufacturers, who are more interested in creating fashions to sell shoes than in providing comfort, and of commercial shoe adapters who, being aware of the universality of foot pain, make hay while the sun shines. As long as the word *orthopedic* is included in advertising, they are assured of happy profits garnered from the long-suffering, gullible public.

This is not to say that everyone who deals with painful feet does not do so with the best of motives; I am sure most do their best. But where can anyone turn to learn about problems of the feet? Many palliative approaches to foot pain are temporarily pain-relieving, but unless proper shoes are available to patients who have been relieved of pain by conservative or surgical means, pain sooner or later surely returns.

Thus we are faced with a vicious circle of cause and effect, and it would be foolhardy to suggest that this work can change the situation as much as I would wish, especially since bespoke shoemakers are a dying breed.

However, it is my hope that some of the knowledge and experience which form the basis of this book may offer those who care for painful feet some new practical ideas which they may incorporate into their practice to bring relief from suffering to a goodly number of patients.

In the preparation of this book I have drawn on the work of many who deserve more credit than I can offer through simple acknowledgment of my gratitude.

Chapter 2, in which anatomy is reviewed, I have taken, with all the illustrations, almost entirely from the *Hand Atlas of Human Anatomy,* 7th Ed., Vol. I, by W. Spalteholz, translated by Lewellys F. Barker, with the cooperation of J. P. Lippincott Co., that claims no copyright interest. The source is gratefully acknowledged.

Chapter 3 is based on discussions with several expert kinesiologists, particularly F. Eugene Miller, R.P.T. Eleanor J. Carlin, R.P.T., Assistant Professor in the School of Allied Medical Sciences at the University of Pennsylvania, added the finishing touches. To these two experts I am especially grateful.

Chapter 4 is culled from multiple sources acknowledged in the bibliography and from experience.

Chapter 5 is taken almost verbatim from my book *Joint Pain — Diagnosis and Treatment Using Manipulative Techniques,* and I am grateful to my publishers, Little, Brown and Company, for their permission to reproduce it.

Chapters 6 through 9 are in the nature of an anthology collected through the years and, again, acknowledgment of the sources is to be found in the bibliography. However, Chapter 9 is based exclusively on the work of my late father James B. Mennell, M.D., and taken from his book *Physical Treatment by Movement and Massage,* J. & A. Churchill Ltd., London. Permission to use this material is gratefully acknowledged.

Chapter 10 comes largely from experience, but the reference to the use of the Vita-Ped is by express permission of its inventor, Earl C. Bullock of Portland, Oregon, who also provided the illustrations for its use. To Mr. Bullock I extend my gratitude. Subsequently the Vita-Ped Company which now owns the rights added its permission.

Chapters 11 and 12 result from preceptorship training by my father and our bespoke shoemaker, R. J. Thomas of London, who succeeds Rowley and Sons. The Mennell family's association with these remarkable artists (or, if you will, craftsmen) stretches over three generations. Mr. Thomas corrected the manuscript of these chapters and deserves credit for valuable contributions to them.

A portion of Chapter 12 is based on the work of Emil D. W. Hauser, M.D., of Chicago, who has very kindly given me his permission to quote extensively and reproduce an illustration from his paper "Management of Lesions of the Subtalar Joint," *Surgical Clinics of North America,* February, 1945, Chicago Number, which makes reference to his book *Diseases of the Foot.* To Dr. Hauser and to W. B. Saunders Company I extend my gratitude.

I am especially indebted to my friend Roger Shannon, M.D., whom I conned into using his great avocational talents to produce the line drawings, in spite of his dearth of spare time and to the deprivation of his family and busy radiological practice.

For the original photography I am greatly indebted to Matthew Kahn, clinical photographer at the Philadelphia General Hospital, whose excellence of work speaks for itself. Most of the x-rays are taken from the Department of Radiology of the Philadelphia General Hospital, and I am grateful to George Wohl, M.D., Chief of Radiology, for his permission to use this material. Drs. Stuart Lewis and Mary Powell also made available certain x-rays of their patients about whom we consulted, and my gratitude is extended to them.

For preliminary editing of the original manuscript, I cannot adequately thank Audrie Bobb, M.D., John Lenox, a potential consumer at the end of his fourth year at the Medical School of the University of Pennsylvania, H. Breffni O'Neill, M.D., and Jerry R. Hughes, M.D., also potential consumers. They spent many hours clarifying what might otherwise have remained obscure to the reader.

For the original typescript I owe thanks to Mary Evelyn de Nissoff of Pinehurst, North Carolina, who put aside all other work for two weeks to produce a workable manuscript, and this without any medical secretarial background. Mary Van Benschoten, my coordinator, and Margaret Mulholland, my secretary, then produced the final manuscript in their spare time, yet to schedule, and it is difficult adequately to thank them.

James Cook, R.P.T., most generously modeled for almost all the new illustrations, and Bruce McCaleb, R.P.T., modeled for and provided the ballet illustrations. Tim Dorsey, of international surfing fame, provided the illustration of "surfers' foot" and information regarding problems related to the condition.

For help with the index I am greatly indebted to Paul Guarnère and Joseph Van Horn of Westwood, California.

Finally, I acknowledge with deep gratitude the understanding and patience of Mr. Fred Belliveau, General Manager of the Medical Division of Little, Brown and Company, who encouraged me to persevere with the production of this work and extended the deadline for its completion by eighteen months in spite of my contractural obligation.

If I have omitted any due gratitude to anyone, I ask their forgiveness. I hope that all will share any credit this work may deserve and the gratitude of any who benefit from its content. Foot comfort is the foundation of bodily freedom. Foot gear is the foundation of foot comfort. Freedom from foot pain largely allows the pursuit of happiness, an inalienable right, which we as physicians can help others to achieve with more sedulous attention to the cause and treatment of their painful feet.

J. McM. M.

Contents

FOOT PAIN

1

Preamble

Foot pain is ubiquitous, and there is a corresponding wealth of writing on the subject, for the most part from the surgical point of view. The little that has been written from any other approach is largely concerned with foot supports and "surgical" or "corrective" shoes; only a small part of this mass of literature is concerned with remedial and corrective foot exercises.

Dr. Harry C. Stein, of New York, in 1954 wrote: "The preservation of function of the foot, including the design of the shoe for the normal foot, is primarily the responsibility of the orthopaedic surgeon." Yet in 1939, fifteen years earlier, the Judicial Council of the American Medical Association issued an edict saying: ". . . Podiatrists and Chiropodists serve a useful purpose in a field considered not important enough for a Doctor of Medicine to attend and therefore too often neglected." This Council reported podiatry to be "a practice related to medicine in a way similar to dentistry, pharmacy and nursing" and stated further: "General opinion seems to be that Chiropody fairly well satisfies a gap in medical care that the professional has failed to fill."

Ten years later Marcus Kohl, M.D., then Commissioner of Health for New York City, is reported by Stein to have said ". . . it is evident that podiatry has grown out of a definite need for the care of certain conditions of the feet which have been slighted or neglected by the medical practitioner . . . it was inevitable that there would arise a demand for *the talents of professional men* [italics added] who would interest themselves in these and *scores of associated conditions* [italics added] which affect the lower extremities. . . . The podiatrist of today is a professional man *possessed of highly technical knowledge and skills, thoroughly trained and qualified to participate in the practice of medical and surgical acts* [italics added] and in his own field to bring relief and comfort to mankind."

Were it not for the podiatrist, the many patients suffering from foot pain would have difficulty in finding a professional, competent person to whom to turn for relief. The orthopedist, more than anyone else, should have a concern for the extremity; but all too often the foot problem is left untreated by him unless the particular difficulty might be solved by surgical intervention; and even surgery, when indicated, is frequently only part of the answer to a pain problem. Were it not for the podiatrist, the patient would be left to the mercy of commercial devices in his search for relief — and all too often these "devices" are expensive, ineffectual, and even harmful. But in the United States there are less than ten thousand practicing, trained podiatrists to help man stand on his own two feet with as little discomfort as possible. In general, the physician, with the exception of the occasional specialist in physical medicine and orthopedist, is not trained to accomplish this task.

The public looks to the medical profession to care for its ills, be they of visceral or of musculoskeletal origin. Physicians should not be satisfied to accept the fact that such a common problem as foot pain is "fairly well cared for" by anyone less well trained than themselves — especially when, as suggested by Dr. Kohl, foot problems are the basis of "scores of associated conditions . . . ," which is certainly the truth.

To whom should this work be addressed? Because there are indeed scores of conditions causing foot pain which are easily mistaken for local foot problems and treated as such, a patient may have treatment of the real problem delayed to his detriment; for this reason, this should be a book for physicians. If so, the podiatrist may well be offended, as it is on record that the medical profession has neglected this field. If it is written for podiatrists, physicians may take offense as it is clearly a medical textbook slanted particularly at differential diagnosis of causes of musculo-skeletal pain, with special reference to the feet. The orthopedist may then object and claim that it is not a textbook at all because the book almost entirely ignores the surgical approach to the treatment of foot pain.

A textbook on foot pain should include a discussion on as many of the causes of pain in the foot as possible; in this work an attempt is made to do this. But in so doing, a very special effort is made to limit the discussion to the causes of foot pain due to factual, underlying pathological processes rather than to spurious diagnoses such as the sinus tarsi syndrome, postural foot pain, and the flat foot.

A detailed review of anatomy is not considered necessary in a work such as this for the answers to foot pain cannot be found in the study of the dead foot. The anatomy of the foot is best de-scribed in the classic textbooks on anatomy and is best read in the original works. A short review is presented in Chapter 2 not to be studied for the sake of anatomy but to remind the reader of the great complexity of the foot, its function, and its state of being.

Again, many excellent accounts of congenital problems of the feet are readily available to the reader. Since they are compre-hensive in their presentation and deal efficiently with the various problems, nothing is to be gained by secondhand, repetitious work in this area.

A textbook should offer a specific form of treatment for every pathological condition that may underlie pain in the foot, but in this work the discussion of treatment is limited to those conditions that respond to methods of physical treatment, support, and special shoes. It does not cover exercise therapy as a treatment of foot pain; this approach to the problem cannot be very successful or, if only because of its ease of prescription and execution, such an approach would already have found universal acceptance.

A textbook would have to include a review of and much detail of an enormous amount of orthopedic literature which is better written by the original authors. That so many operative procedures have been devised and then modified suggests, in itself, that the answer to foot pain is frequently not to be found in the orthopedic surgical approach.

A textbook should review foot supports, shoe modifications, and shoe making. The fact that supports are commercially mass produced suggests either that there is no need to enlarge on this topic, or that what is known about them leaves much to be desired. It is hoped, however, that the chapter on foot supports will present something new. Shoe modifications in the treatment of feet are better dealt with in the original writings and do not contribute sufficiently to the relief of foot pain to warrant a detailed review. It was frustrating to write the chapter on shoe making because there are so few shoe makers to be found in the United States and bespoke shoe making is almost a dead art.

So, though much of what is to be presented may not be original, it is practical and is based on experience in treating patients who have suffered from foot pain that continued in spite of wearing conventional (and sometimes unconventional) supports, in spite of doing exercises, in spite of minor and major surgery, in spite of wearing expensive "orthopedic" and other "surgical" shoes, and in spite of expensive and varied methods of conventional pedicare. It is hoped that this experience may help *all* those concerned with patients who suffer from foot pain of the common, everyday variety.

2

Anatomy

Most surgical procedures carried out for relief of foot pain are designed in some way or another to alter the "mechanics" of the foot. These designs may aim at reconstruction, correction, or destruction. The frontispiece reproduces x-rays of the feet of a 42-year-old woman who at the age of 18 had normal, painless feet. Four years later painful bunions had developed. The destruction of her bones and joints resulted from three different surgical procedures, each carried out for the relief of pain. Today, she is about to undergo a fourth surgical procedure because the foot pain is worse than ever. These feet are beyond correction or reconstruction; only further destruction is contemplated.

For the most part operations are designed from anatomical studies made on the dead foot. Anatomists have perpetuated misconceptions of function because of their preoccupation with the dead rather than the living. This perhaps is less true when dealing with muscles than with joints, but as muscles cannot function normally unless the joints upon which they act move normally, there is little merit to knowing a great deal about the function of one structure without knowing as much about the function of the other. In addition, there is the problem of pain, and there is no way of telling by cadaver dissection either in the anatomy laboratory or in the postmortem room whether or not a morphological change has been responsible for pain in life. A similar problem is faced by radiologists who, in problems of the musculoskeletal system, can report only seeing the abnormal shadows of anatomical change without discussing their significance in relation to a patient's complaints. Cineradiography should materially add to our knowledge of living joint function before too long.

Furthermore, to the anatomist, a foot is a foot. No patient, however, has two identical feet. He may have pain in both feet, but the cause may be different in each. The commercial shoemaker also ignores the disparity between two feet in a single individual.

The basis of most anatomical teaching about the feet is centered on the suggestion that a foot architecturally is designed about two arches — the longitudinal arch (sometimes divided into two) and the transverse arch — and that there is a tripod of weight bearing: posteriorly on the calcaneus and anteriorly on the heads of the first and fifth metatarsal bones. This classic concept should be honored more as fiction than as fact.

That there are arches in the feet is indisputable, but that their variance from normal causes pain is most often misleading. There is, however, an important and ill-supported arch at the bases of the metatarsal bones, strong at the apex but weak laterally, which is easily strained and is a potent source of pain. It is necessary only to look at the shape of any group of painless feet (Fig. 2-1) to appreciate the wide variability of normal. A very large number of patients who suffer from foot pain offer for examination a foot or feet with apparently perfectly normal arches, while, conversely, many people with apparently grossly abnormal arches are free of foot pain.

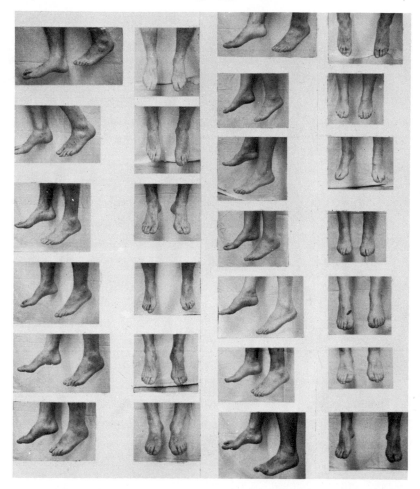

FIGURE 2-1. Thirteen pairs of feet all of which are clinically pain-free, i.e., "normal." Each pair is shown from the front and from the side. Variation in shape and size has little relation to symptoms of foot pain.

Bones

The anatomical arches of the foot largely depend on the architectural design of the bones that go to make them up; this can well be appreciated by looking at a demonstration skeleton (Figs. 2-2, 2-3, and 2-4).

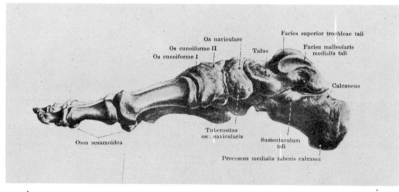

A

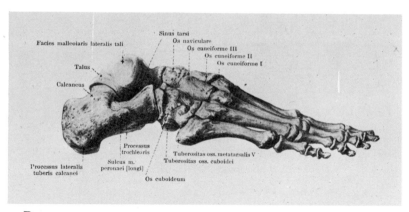

B

FIGURE 2-2.   Medial (A) and lateral (B) views of the skeleton of the foot. See also Figures 2-3 and 2-4. The "arches" are architecturally sound in design, except at the bases of the metatarsal bones. This supports the suggestion that it is futile to attempt their correction once growth is completed — that is, in the adult.

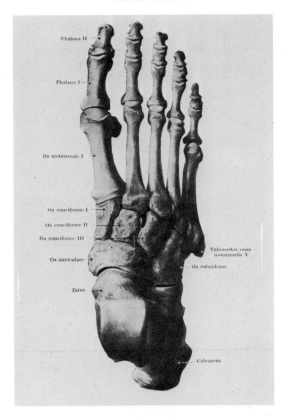

FIGURE 2-3.   Dorsal view of the skeleton of the foot.

With constant wear and tear and overloading, the architectural stability alone might break down. The bones are spared this because the junctions between them are protected by the normal anatomical structures that form and support any synovial joint. The ligaments that reinforce the synovial capsules are plentiful and strong, and the architectural stability is further enhanced by the tendons of the extrinsic muscles, the presence of intrinsic muscles, the tough plantar fascia, and the rather specialized integument of the foot. There are in a foot 26 bones and 30 major synovial joints to be considered antomically if one counts the

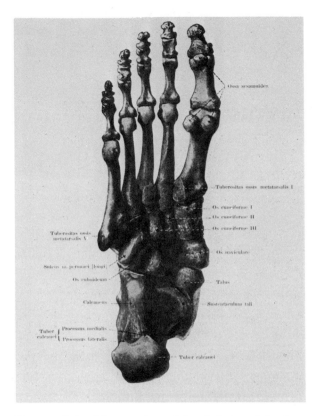

FIGURE 2-4.   Plantar view of the skeleton of the foot.

subtalar joint and the mortise joint each as a single joint even though they are both multiple-faceted joints, if one includes the joints between the bases of the metatarsals while counting the tarsal-metatarsal articulations, and if one excludes the junctions between the heads of the metatarsal bones, which behave like joints although they are not. A pathological condition in any one of these joints may be the cause of foot pain. Commonly there are two sesamoid bones under the head of the first metatarsal bone, and occasionally a third sesamoid bone is found proximal to the medial aspect of the navicula.

The shape and positioning of the three cuneiform bones are perfections of architecture, the second cuneiform being the keystone. Its sloping sides lock the three cuneiforms into a bridge, the second cuneiform absorbing forces from all directions. The second metatarsal bone locks into a mortise made up of the anterior parts of the first and third cuneiform bones medially and laterally, with the second cuneiform proximally affording additional architectural stability. It is of passing interest that only in man is there a consistent metatarsophalangeal joint forming the ball of the foot.

Ligaments

The system of supportive joint ligaments in the ankle and foot is extremely complex, as is well illustrated in Figures 2-5 through 2-8. It is not necessary for the physician to know the exact attachment, insertion, and name of each ligament as long as he remembers what a normal ligament feels like, the location of the major palpable ligaments, and the fact that ligaments are *never* tender on palpation unless they are sprained or torn, or — and this is most important — unless there is something wrong with the joint that the ligament supports. If there is tenderness on palpation of a ligament, there is always something wrong. The major ligaments of diagnostic importance are discussed below.

DELTOID LIGAMENT.   The deltoid ligament is the medial collateral ligament of the "ankle" and is divided into four main bands (Fig. 2-5). From the posterior aspect forward these are the posterior talotibial ligament, the main calcaneotibial ligament, the anterior talotibial ligament, and the tibionavicular ligament. Although the anterior fibers of the deltoid ligament support the

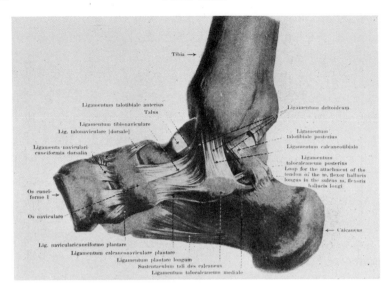

FIGURE 2-5.   Complex arrangement of supporting ligaments of the foot and ankle from the medial aspect. See also Figures 2-3 and 2-4.

talonavicular joint, to all intents and purposes tenderness on palpation of it, in the absence of ligament trauma, most often indicates a pathological problem of the mortise joint.

LATERAL COLLATERAL LIGAMENT.   This ligament is divided into three main bands (Fig. 2-6): posteriorly, the posterior talofibular ligament; centrally, the main calcaneofibular ligament; and anteriorly, the anterior talofibular ligament. Tenderness on palpation of any part of this ligament, in the absence of ligament trauma, also indicates a pathological problem of the mortise joint.

Tenderness on palpation of the anterior talofibular fibers of the lateral collateral ligament must never be confused with palpatory tenderness in the sinus tarsi. The sinus tarsi, being a hole, cannot have a pathological problem in it, but at its base is the only clinically palpable ligament of the subtalar joint.

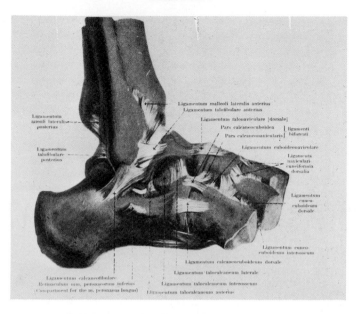

FIGURE 2-6.   Supporting ligaments of the foot and ankle from the
lateral aspect.

LATERAL TALOCALCANEAL LIGAMENT.   This is the ligament
(Fig. 2-6) that is palpated through the sinus tarsi. When tender,
in the absence of ligament strain, a pathological condition is
present in the subtalar joint. This is one of the most important
signs that may be elicited on clinical examination of the "ankle,"
and its significance is often overlooked or misinterpreted as being
evidence of the nebulous "sinus tarsi syndrome."

DORSAL TALONAVICULAR LIGAMENT.   This ligament (Figs.
2-5, 2-6, and 2-8A) is not clinically well differentiated, yet
tenderness on palpation over the talonavicular joint probably
arises from it. The area merits palpation for purposes of differential diagnosis of the location of a pathological process causing
symptoms.

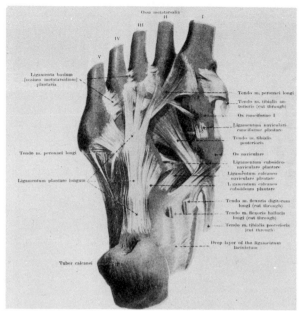

A

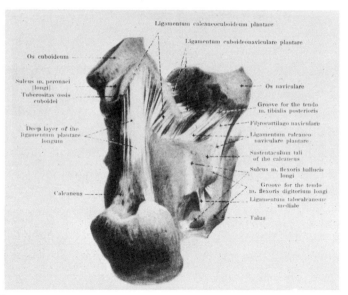

B

FIGURE 2-7.   Supporting ligaments of the foot from the plantar
aspect. A. Superficial layer. B. Deep layer.

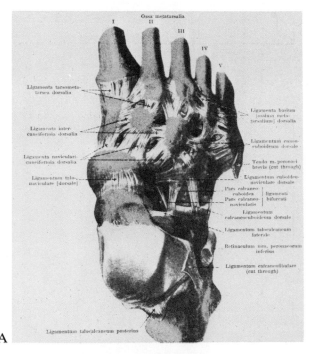

A

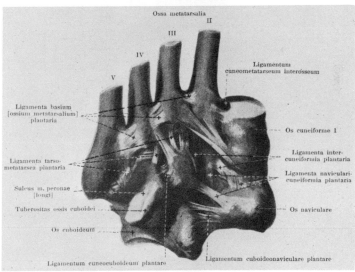

B

FIGURE 2-8.   A. Supporting ligaments of the foot from the dorsal aspect. B. The deep layer of supporting ligaments of the foot from the plantar aspect.

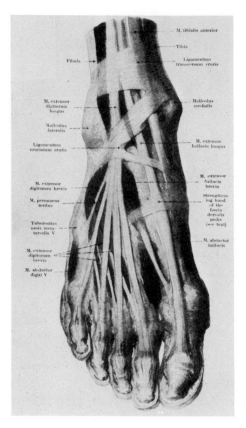

FIGURE 2-9.   The dorsum of the foot showing the retinacula confining the long extensor muscle tendons as they cross over the ankle from the lower leg into the foot.

LONG PLANTAR LIGAMENT.   This is a nonspecific joint-supporting ligament stretching from the plantar calcaneal tubercle forward across the plantar aspect of the cuboid laterally, with its medial fibers passing forward across the third cuneiform bone, inserting into a ligamentous aponeurosis at the bases of the second, third, and fourth metatarsal bones (Figs. 2-7 and 2-8). Calcaneocuboid joint disorders give rise to tenderness of this ligament, but it is situated deep below the skin with many structures overlying it. Tenderness from it is difficult to differentiate from plantar fascia pain on clinical examination.

RETINACULA.   At the ankle, both laterally and medially, and also over the most distal part of the lower leg and over the most proximal aspect of the dorsum of the foot there are retinacula which confine the extrinsic muscle tendons, blood vessels, and nerves as they pass from the lower leg into the foot. There is a superior peroneal and an inferior peroneal retinaculum, a superior tibial and an inferior tibial retinaculum, and a superior and inferior extensor retinaculum. Trauma with resulting edema and maybe tenosynovitis, where tendon sheaths are present, cause pressure problems on all these structures, with symptoms of entrapment. The retinacula on the dorsal aspect of the foot are shown in Figures 2-9 through 2-12.

Muscles

The muscles that act upon the foot are divided into two main groups: the extrinsic muscles and the intrinsic muscles.

Extrinsic Muscles.   The extrinsic muscles, except for the gastrocnemius muscle, take their origin in the leg below the knee. For convenience they are divided into three groups: (1) those in the anterior compartment; (2) those in the lateral compartment; and (3) those in the posterior compartment.

ANTERIOR COMPARTMENT MUSCLES.   The muscles of the anterior compartment are the tibialis anterior, the extensor digitorum longus, and the extensor hallucis longus (Fig. 2-10).
The *tibialis anterior* takes its origin from the lateral tibial

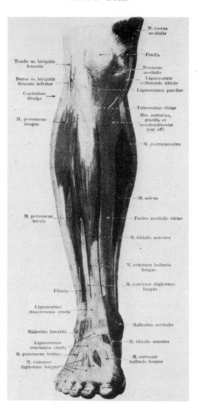

FIGURE 2-10. The extrinsic muscles of the anterior compartment of the lower leg. These are the tibialis anterior, the extensor digitorum longus, and the extensor hallucis longus.

condyle and from the proximal half of the anterolateral aspect of the tibia. After crossing to the inner side of the ankle, the muscle inserts under the base of the first metatarsal bone and medial cuneiform bone. While acting as a dorsiflexor and invertor of the foot, its braking action against body weightbearing on flexion of the knee is far more demanding and as important.

The *extensor digitorum longus* arises from the lateral condyle of the tibia and from the upper anterior surface of the fibula and divides into four insertions, one each on the dorsal surface of phalanges of the four lateral toes. The muscle has a dual function of extending these toes and also of assisting in dorsiflexion of the ankle.

The *extensor hallucis longus* arises from the midportion of the fibula anteriorly. It is inserted on the dorsal aspect of the base of the distal phalanx of the big toe. It has a dual action of extending the big toe and assisting dorsiflexion of the ankle.

LATERAL COMPARTMENT MUSCLES. The muscles of the lateral compartment are the peroneus longus, the peroneus brevis, and the peroneus tertius (Fig. 2-11).

The *peroneus longus* arises from the lateral aspect of the lateral condyle of the tibia and from the upper part of the shaft of the fibula. Its tendon passes behind the lateral malleolus of the fibula, where it shares a tendon sheath with the brevis and is maintained in position by a retinaculum. It passes across the sole of the foot to insert on the first cuneiform bone and on the base of the first metatarsal bone on their plantar aspects. Its action is eversion of the foot and plantar flexion of the ankle.

The *peroneus brevis* arises from the lower lateral aspect of the shaft of the fibula and its tendon, together with the tendon of the peroneus longus, whose sheath it shares, passes under the retinaculum behind the lateral malleolus, but, instead of crossing the foot from its lateral to its medial aspect as does the longus, it passes forward to insert on the dorsal aspect of the base of the fifth metatarsal bone. Its action is chiefly that of eversion of the foot, and it assists plantar flexion.

The *peroneus tertius* arises from the lower part of the shaft of the fibula but more anteriorly than the peroneus longus or brevis. Its tendon passes in front of the lateral malleolus under the ex-

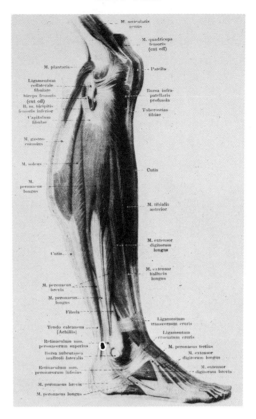

FIGURE 2-11.   The extrinsic muscles of the lateral compartment of
the lower leg. These are the peroneus longus, the peroneus brevis,
and the peroneus tertius.

tensor retinacula to be inserted on the dorsal aspect of the mid-
shaft of the fifth metatarsal bone. Its action assists in dorsiflexion
and eversion of the foot.

POSTERIOR COMPARTMENT MUSCLES.   The muscles of the
posterior compartment are divided into a superficial group and a
deep group. The superficial group is composed of the plantaris
muscle, the gastrocnemius muscle, and the soleus muscle (Fig. 2-
12). The deep group consists of the flexor digitorum longus, the

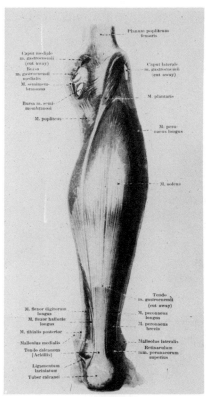
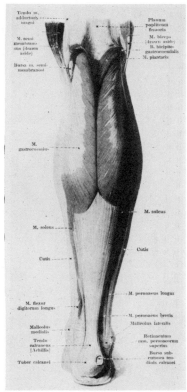

A   B

FIGURE 2-12. A and B. The superficial extrinsic muscles of the posterior compartment of the lower leg: the plantaris muscle, the gastrocnemius muscle, and the soleus muscle.

flexor hallucis longus, and the tibialis posterior muscles (Fig. 2-13).

The *gastrocnemius muscle* arises from each of the condyles of the femur posteriorly, and the *soleus muscle* arises from the proximal posterior aspects of both the tibia and the fibula. These muscles have a common insertion, as they form the Achilles tendon which inserts into the posterior aspect of the calcaneus. The action of these two muscles is to plantar flex the foot at the

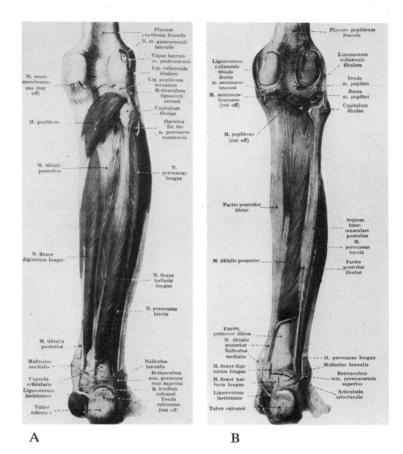

FIGURE 2-13.   A and B. The deep extrinsic muscles of the posterior
compartment of the lower leg: the flexor digitorum longus, the flexor
hallucis longus, and the tibialis posterior.

mortise joint. The *plantaris muscle* is a vestigial part of the
soleus-gastrocnemius complex. Its clinical significance far ex-
ceeds its anatomical importance.

In the deep group, the *flexor digitorum longus* takes its origin
from the posterior aspect of the shaft of the tibia and passes down
the posteromedial part of the leg. Its tendon, encased in a sheath,
passes under the tibial retinacula behind the medial malleolus

to divide into four separate tendons which pass obliquely across the plantar aspect of the foot, each tendon being inserted into the terminal phalanx of each of the four lateral toes. The action of this muscle is not only to plantar flex the toes but also to assist inversion of the foot.

The *flexor hallucis longus* takes its origin from the lower part of the posterior aspect of the fibula and passes downward on the posterolateral aspect of the lower leg where its tendon, encased in a sheath and retained by the tibial retinacula, passes around the medial malleolus in a groove on the calcaneus forward to insert on the distal phalanx of the big toe. Its action, besides plantar flexing the big toe, also helps to invert the foot. Great strain is laid on this tendon if the ankle is pronated, and there is a tendency for the medial side of the foot to flatten.

The *tibialis posterior* takes its origin from the upper third of the tibia and perhaps two-thirds of the fibula and from the interosseus membrane between them. The muscle passes down the leg posterior to the tibia to form its tendon which, in its sheath, passes around the medial malleolus, encased in the medial retinacula, to insert on the undersurface of the navicula with tendinous slips to other tarsal and metatarsal bones. It assists in foot inversion, adduction, plantar flexion, and in supporting the architectural features of the whole tarsus.

Intrinsic Muscles.   The intrinsic muscles, with the exception of the extensor digitorum brevis (and extensor hallucis brevis) and four dorsal interosseus muscles, are all situated in the plantar aspect of the foot.

Dorsal Intrinsic Muscles.   The *extensor digitorum brevis* and *extensor hallucis brevis* take their origin from the lateral and superior surfaces of the calcaneus in front of the sinus tarsi. They divide into four bellies and tendons which pass forward and medially. The lateral three tendons fuse with the corresponding tendons of the extensor digitorum longus and insert into the second and third phalanges of the second, third, and fourth toes; the medial and largest portion of the muscle, which is now called the extensor hallucis brevis, attaches to the base of the first phalanx of the great toe.

There are four *dorsal interosseus* muscles which take their origin from the adjacent sides of each pair of the metatarsal bones and insert at the lateral aspects of the bases of the second, third, and fourth proximal phalanges. It should be noted that the first dorsal interosseus muscle takes its origin from the bases of the first and second metatarsal bones and that the proximal phalanx of the second toe gives insertion medially to the first dorsal interosseus and laterally to the second dorsal interosseus muscles (Fig. 2-14).

PLANTAR INTRINSIC MUSCLES.   The plantar intrinsic muscles are commonly described in three layers — superficial, middle, and deep. In the most superficial layer are the abductor hallucis, the flexor digitorum brevis, and the abductor digiti quinti (Fig. 2-15). The *abductor hallucis* takes its origin from the tuber calcanei, from the deltoid ligament, and from the navicular bone and inserts in the base of the proximal phalanx of the big toe. The *flexor digitorum brevis* takes its origin from the medial aspect of the undersurface of the calcaneus and from the plantar fascia. It divides into four muscle bellies and tendons which insert into the middle phalanges of the second, third, fourth, and fifth toes after decussating to allow the tendons of the flexor digitorum longus to pass between the medial and lateral parts of each tendon. The *abductor digiti quinti* takes its origin from the inferior surfaces of the calcaneus lateral to the origin of the flexor digitorum brevis as well as from the plantar fascia. It passes

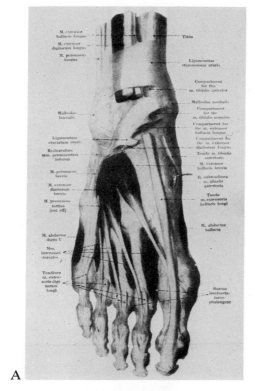

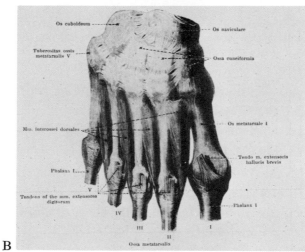

FIGURE 2-14. The dorsal intrinsic muscles. These are (A) the extensor hallucis brevis and extensor digitorum brevis, and (B) four dorsal interosseus muscles.

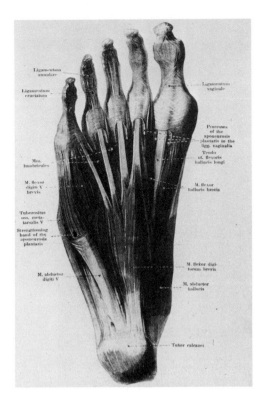

FIGURE 2-15. The superficial layer of the plantar intrinsic muscles: the flexor digitorum brevis and the abductor digiti quinti.

forward and laterally to insert into the inferior aspect of the
base of the proximal phalanx of the fifth toe.

The muscles of the middle layer in the plantar aspect of the
foot are the quadratus plantae and the lumbrical muscles (Fig.
2-16). The *quadratus plantae* takes its origin from the inferior
and medial surfaces of the calcaneus and passes forward to insert
in the lateral margin of the tendon of the flexor digitorum longus.
The *lumbrical muscles* take their origin partly from the medial
margin and partly from the opposed margins of the tendons of
the flexor digitorum longus. They then insert into the medial

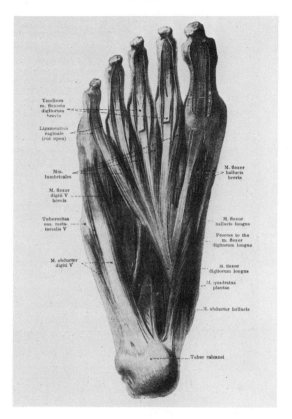

FIGURE 2-16.   The middle layer of the plantar intrinsic muscles:
the quadratus plantae and the lumbricales.

surfaces of the proximal phalanges of the second, third, fourth,
and fifth toes.

The deep layer of intrinsic muscles in the plantar aspect are
the flexor hallucis brevis, the adductor hallucis (Fig. 2-17), and
the interossei (Fig. 2-18). The *flexor hallucis brevis* takes its
origin from the plantar surface of the cuneiform bones and the
navicular bone and divides into two tendinous insertions which
run to the two sesamoid bones and to the base of the proximal
phalanx of the great toe.

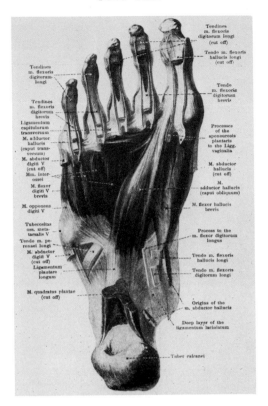

FIGURE 2-17. The deep layer of the plantar intrinsic muscles: the flexor hallucis brevis and the adductor hallucis.

The *adductor hallucis* takes its origin from two heads. The oblique head arises from the bases of the metatarsal bones two through four, from the third cuneiform, and from the cuboid. The muscle converges into one insertion into the lateral aspect of the lateral sesamoid bone and the base of the proximal phalanx of the big toe. The transverse part of the muscle takes its origin from the capsular ligaments of the metatarsophalangeal joints of the second, third, fourth, and fifth toes and inserts into the lateral sesamoid bone and base of the proximal phalanx of the great toe.

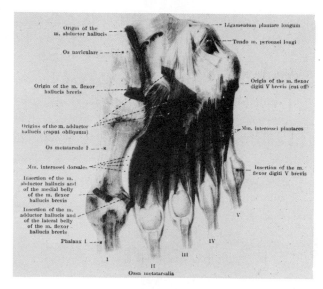

FIGURE 2-18.   The plantar interosseus muscles.

The interosseus muscles are considered together with the flexor digiti quinti brevis and the opponens digiti quinti (Fig. 2-18). There are *three interosseus muscles* on the plantar aspect of the foot; they take their origins from the medial surfaces of the third, fourth, and fifth metatarsal bones and insert on the medial aspect of the proximal phalangeal bones of the third, fourth, and fifth toes, also joining the tendons of the extensor digitorum muscles.

The *flexor digiti quinti brevis* originates from the base of the fifth metatarsal bone and inserts in the base of the proximal phalanx of the fifth toe.

The *opponens digiti quinti* takes its origin from the long plantar ligament and from the flexor digitorum quinti brevis and inserts in the distal part of the lateral aspect of the fifth metatarsal bone.

Tendon Sheaths

The tendon sheaths of the muscles of the foot are much more complicated than those of the hand. Up to this point only the common tendon sheath of the peroneus longus and brevis has been referred to. The peroneus longus has a subsequent tendon sheath as it crosses obliquely across the plantar aspect of the foot. The posterior tibial muscle has a tendon sheath which passes

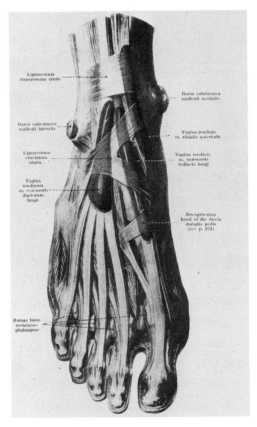

FIGURE 2-19.   Arrangement of the tendon sheaths around the ankle and in the foot on the dorsal aspect. See Figures 2-20 and 2-21.

behind the medial malleolus and ends at the navicular bone. The
flexor digitorum longus has a tendon sheath which begins posterior to the medial malleolus and ends at the level of the navicular
bone. The flexor hallucis longus has a tendon sheath which also
starts posterior to the medial malleolus and finishes beneath the
navicular bone. These three tendons and their sheaths are retained by a retinaculum which passes from beneath the medial
malleolus and inserts on the calcaneus. Then there are five tendon
sheaths invaginating the flexor tendons of the toes which start
proximal to the heads of the metatarsal bones and progress as far
as the bases of the middle phalanx in each toe. On the dorsum of
the foot there is a tendon sheath invaginating the tendon of the
extensor digitorum longus muscle, the extensor hallucis longus
muscle, and the tendon of the tibialis anterior. Figures 2-19, 2-
20, and 2-21 illustrate the arrangement of the tendon sheaths.

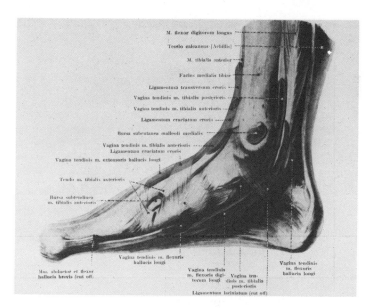

FIGURE 2-20.   Tendon sheaths around the ankle and in the foot
on the medial aspect.

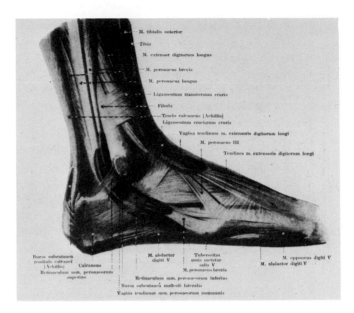

FIGURE 2-21.   Tendon sheaths around the ankle and in the foot
on the lateral aspect.

Bursae

The bursae in the foot are the Achilles or posterior calcaneal
bursa, the subcalcaneal bursa, the intermetatarsal head bursae,
the lumbrical bursae, and the bursae on the medial aspect of
the metatarsophalangeal joint of the big toe and the lateral aspect
of the metatarsophalangeal joint of the little toe. There are also
subcutaneous bursae over both malleoli at the ankle. Figures 2-
11, 2-12B, 2-19, 2-20, and 2-21 show many of the bursae of
the foot.

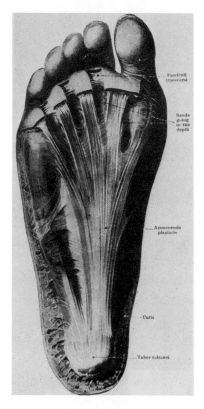

FIGURE 2-22.   The plantar fascia of the foot.

Plantar Fascia

The plantar fascia (Fig. 2-22) covers the inferior surface of
the muscles of the sole of the foot. It takes its origin from the
tuberosity of the calcaneus and extends forward to insert in five
separate processes into the sole of the foot. Intramuscular septa
also enter into the depths of the foot to insert into various inter-
stitial structures.

3

Function of the Foot

The foot has three basic functions: (1) support, which includes posture; (2) propulsion, which includes gait and dexterity; and (3) dexterity — not only the dexterity of ambulation but also that which is intrinsic and is usually developed only in people without hands. If these functions are performed correctly, pain will not develop in the normal foot — at least not until the foot is encased in an ill-designed shoe.

The foot is almost as beautifully designed as the hand. Indeed, people without hands, especially if their absence is congenital, train their feet to substitute for their hands in the most remarkably efficient and useful manner.

Certainly, we should be as clumsy as apes, and possibly more helpless, if we paid as little attention to our hands as we do to our feet. If we encased our hands in hand-shoes for most of our lives as we do our feet, the dextrous functions of the extrinsic and intrinsic muscles of the hands would soon be lost. If the muscles lose their function, the joints rapidly lose their movement; elastic tissue in muscle, ligament, and capsule is lost to be replaced by fibrous tissue, which in the end results in contractures, deformities, and uselessness.

Forces Transmitted to the Feet.   H. R. Quinby, in his book *Pacemakers of Progress,* estimates that the cumulative force to which each foot is subjected during a day is the equivalent of 704 tons in a person weighing 200 pounds who is estimated to walk 8 miles a day. The structures of the foot can withstand this enormous daily work load with comparative comfort and freedom from the overt pathological changes that usually result from trauma because of the architectural perfection of the bones, joints, ligaments, muscles, fascia, protective bursae, and skin, and because the force is dissipated by the perfect use of the mechanical properties and principles of elasticity, fulcrums, and levers. These structures could not survive without similar mechanical perfection in the use of all the rest of the musculoskeletal structures, without the perfect working of all the neuromuscular mechanisms, and without their perfect nourishment by the vascular and lymphatic systems. To think of feet only as feet is intellectually dishonest. More is the pity that physicians have given up the study and care of most patients with foot problems.

Keystone to Foot Function

"ARCHES" AND THEIR VARIATIONS. Probably the best example of the perfectly functioning foot is that of the expertly trained ballet dancer. In the *first position* (Fig. 3-1A) the feet appear to be flat. In the performance of the *dégagé derrière* (Fig. 3-1B) the left (front) foot retains its flat appearance, whereas the back foot now shows a perfect arch (Fig. 3-2C). (The feet illustrated belong to the same model.) Freedom from pain in the feet is a prerequisite to ballet dancing. Flat-footedness is an ethnic characteristic of the Negro, who seldom complains of foot pain, as compared with the less flat-footed Caucasian who frequently does.

If one persists in stressing deviations of the arches from normal

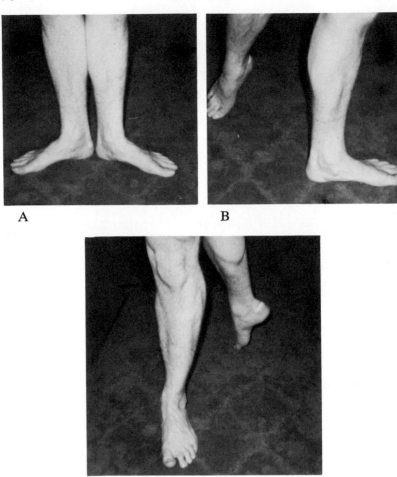

A   B

C

FIGURE 3-1.   The apparent flatness of the feet in the ballet dancer
as he adopts the *first position* (A). B. View of the same dancer
showing the seeming flatness of the left foot as he adopts the position of the *dégagé derrière*. C. Perfect arch of right foot of same
dancer in same position. Compare B and C.

as being the primary cause of foot pain, then it is reasonable to regard the tarsal navicular bone — the keystone of the major longitudinal arch — as the seat of the pain. Yet the navicular bone is seldom considered to undergo pathological changes except when there is a congenital bar, said to be a cause of congenital spastic flatfoot, or when it is the seat of osteochondritis juvenilis (Köhler's disease). It is not even common to see the radiological diagnosis of osteoarthritis in the joints in which the navicula is involved. The talonavicular joint is destroyed in the surgical procedure of triple arthrodesis when performed as a "stabilizing" procedure, but in operations done for pain in this area the more selective subastragaloid (subtalar) fusion is usually sufficient. That the triple arthrodesis is performed for the relief of pain more likely suggests the inability of the surgeon clinically to distinguish from which joint of three the pain is arising.

THE TALUS.   If the role of arches is less stressed, then it becomes apparent that the talus is the keystone to normal function of the foot — indeed, it is a unique bone. No muscles are attached to it, and it has four major articulating facets — five if the calcaneotalar facet is regarded in its two separate anatomical parts.

Because no muscles are attached to it, if movement in any of the joints in which it plays a part is lost, no exercise regimen can hope to restore its movement to normal. It is an accepted orthopedic fact that impaired movement is painful movement. Any talar joint movement is a prime example of joint-play movement, the restoration of which, when it is lost or impaired, must be manipulative if function is to be restored and pain relieved. The only alternative treatment of a painful talar joint must be its destruction by fusion. As inversion and eversion take place at

the midtarsal joints and at the subtalar joint, anyone with a subtalar fusion remains almost fully functional for everyday purposes.

Dynamics of Support

The supportive function of the foot is anything but static, and
if one stands motionless on the feet, foot pain ensues in a very
short time. In standing, the muscles of the feet, both intrinsic and
extrinsic, are in a constant state of reciprocal activity and the
joints are constantly adjusting the relationship of the articulating
facets maintaining their normal physiological condition. To stand
in shoes that are too small in any dimension is to suffer almost
immediately.

Posture

Posture and gait are essentially individual characteristics. Both
are functions of the feet, and foot pain may result from either
faulty posture or faulty gait or may cause either of them.

I believe it is impossible to change an individual's inherent
posture, certainly in adult life, and gait training as it is usually
carried out in physical therapy has always seemed to me an awful
waste of a therapist's skill and time. But gait retraining for the
return of dexterity in ambulation is another story and requires a
great deal of skill.

Standing Postural Training. Therapeutic correction of posture, in the treatment of pain problems truly arising from faulty
posture, stretches tightened ligaments and muscles and feels sufficiently strange or uncomfortable to the patient that he may

abandon his treatment. But with perseverance and encouragement from the therapist this should not prove an insurmountable problem, especially if the therapist uses adjunctive therapeutic modalities such as Jacobson's relaxation routine, local ice massage, and relaxing limb massage. Under these circumstances the patient quite rapidly, though still consciously, achieves and maintains his new good habits. It is not long before they become automatic.

If standing is an occupational requirement, foot pain, among other postural pains, may be avoided if attention is paid to the following points. In parenthesis, morbidity following back surgery is decreased by following these simple principles.

STAND WITH FEET APART AT HIP WIDTH.   Standing with the feet apart at hip width enhances lateral balance by decreasing any tendency either to bend to the side or to rotate the lower part of the trunk. This alone then is prophylactic against not only foot pain, because the body weight is distributed equally across the width of both feet, but also against low back pain. This is the position of "at ease" sensibly adopted by the armed forces.

STAND WITH FEET PARALLEL.   If one alternately lifts each foot off the floor and rotates the hip of the elevated leg purely at the hip joint until the foot points straight ahead (the ankle being absolutely relaxed), one becomes aware of the internal hip rotator muscles working and the external rotator muscles being stretched when the foot points forward. Standing with the feet turned out has allowed these muscles to contract, which may be uncomfortable. This position lays abnormal stress on the feet, producing muscle imbalance and ligament strain in them, and painful foot function results (Fig. 3-2).

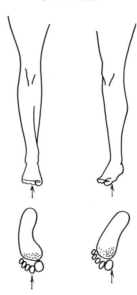

FIGURE 3-2.   *Left:* Correct position of the leg and foot for maximum efficiency of weight bearing and in ambulation. *Right:* What happens when the foot is splayed out and the leg is rotated outward from the hip.

Efforts to correct this must avoid turning in the foot at the ankle and at the tarsal joints. Rotatory correction must come from the hips. Ankle movement is reserved for forward walking (the mortise joint) and for balancing on uneven surfaces (subtalar and midtarsal joints).

Medial rotation of the hip joint elevates the medial border of the foot. Lateral rotation flattens it. This emphasizes the significant relationship of hip joint function to foot function, and to posture and gait. The foot is properly used or abused as the hip directs it, and the cause of pain in the foot may be found in imbalance between the internal and external rotators of the hip.

Similarly, the cause of pain in the foot may be found in the iliotibial band, which, if it is pathologically tight, causes eversion at the ankle and external rotation of the foot. Treatment of the iliotibial band may then be necessary for the relief of foot pain.

STAND WITH KNEES SLIGHTLY FLEXED. Slight flexion of the knee relaxes the gastrocnemius-soleus group of muscles, which in turn relaxes the stresses in the foot in its long axis. The long extrinsic muscles, especially the flexor hallucis longus, also tend to be more relaxed. A relaxed foot must be a resilient foot and therefore a better functioning and painless foot.

STAND WITH PELVIS "ROLLED UNDER." To maintain correct pelvic posture in standing benefits the back more than the feet. However, a tired back makes tired feet, and in posture, as in anything else, one cannot dissociate parts of the body from the whole body. Figure 3-3 illustrates correct pelvic posture and Figure 3-4 incorrect pelvic posture. The correct pelvic posture maintains the normal center of gravity. This decreases the stresses of weight bearing on the feet. To be able to maintain this pelvic

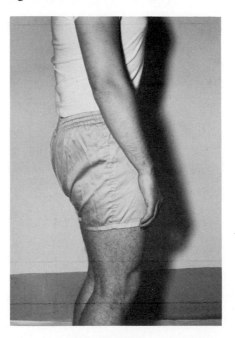

FIGURE 3-3.   Correct posture with the pelvis "rolled under." Compare with Figure 3-4.

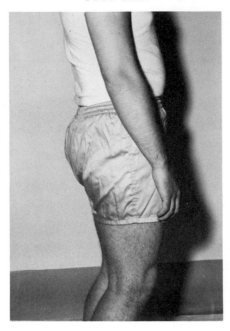

FIGURE 3-4.   Incorrect posture without pelvis "rolled under."

posture, the gluteus maximus muscles and the rectus abdominis muscles must be functioning especially well, so a cause of foot pain, though certainly remote, may be found in lax abdominal muscles. If the knees are not in slight flexion (see above), it is difficult to maintain the pelvis rolled under.

STAND WITH SCAPULAE BRACED AND SHOULDERS PULLED DOWN. Though it may appear that this discussion is becoming less and less concerned with the feet, posture is posture, and any deviation from normal anywhere may affect any part of the musculoskeletal system but especially the feet, which support the whole body. Pelvic and hip postural problems have direct effects on the feet, but the pelvis is attached to the shoulders by the latissimus dorsi muscles. Thus the effect of forequarter posture on the feet may not be so obscure after all.

STAND WITH THE HEAD "AS TALL" AS POSSIBLE AND THE CHIN IN. The head thrust forward with the chin protruding alters the center of gravity of the body and thus unfavorably affects weight bearing on the feet.

Gait

NORMAL (CORRECT) GAIT. As the foot commences its propulsive function after heel strike, which should occur on center (but will be off center if there is ankle pronation), weight bearing progresses forward along the outer aspect of the foot to the head of the fifth metatarsal bone and then fans out across the forefoot, sequentially involving each next metatarsal head until, the leg being carried backward all this time, the foot is ready for "pushoff." At this point the lumbricals and interosseus muscles fix the interphalangeal joints in a reaching and grasping position, and they, assisted by the long toe flexors, fix the forefoot on the floor. The leg is carried backward by the thigh extensors, knee extension being controlled by the quadriceps. The hip muscles rotate the femur outward to an angle (about 30 degrees) that matches the angle of toe flexion at the metatarsophalangeal joints. The gastrocnemius-soleus group then plantar flexes the foot for strong push-off, forcing strong toe extension. Transverse stability of the ankle is preserved by the balanced function of the tibialis anterior, the tibialis posterior, and the peroneus longus and brevis, with assistance from the long flexors and extensors of the toes acting in balance.

ABNORMAL GAITS. One of the commonest gait errors is the same as that in posture — namely, walking with the hip in external rotation. This seriously impairs proper function of the foot to avoid hurting the hip. This gait fault also lays abnormal stresses on the medial collateral ligament of the knee and tends to induce pronation strain of the ankle and flattening of the medial border of the foot. This all adds up to impaired plantar flexion and faulty positioning of the toes, painful weight bearing, and even toe deformity. Correction of these faults occurs with correction of posture and suitable foot exercises (described in Chapter 8).

All these errors can be caused by wearing faulty shoes. Gait analysis must therefore include assessment of the shoes, correction of which may be sufficient by itself to correct the gait problems.

4

Examination

The usual clinical examination of the foot, based as it is upon knowledge gained from the cadaver, does little more than confirm the patient's symptoms and reveal the presence of any variations from a preconceived "normal" that each individual examiner has learned, depending upon how much or how little he has to do with foot problems. If abnormalities are noted in the x-ray, these are seized upon as revealing the cause of the patient's pain. Sometimes laboratory data reveal abnormalities suggesting certain disease processes such as gout and rheumatoid arthritis, and then they become hooks on which diagnosticians hang their hats while very often the true cause of the patient's symptoms is overlooked.

This type of pseudoscientific examination of this part of the musculoskeletal system also results in such meaningless diagnoses as sinus tarsi syndrome, metatarsalgia, calcaneal spur, hallux valgus or rigidus, or perhaps the even less satisfactory diagnosis of osteoarthritis. These diagnoses are certainly descriptive, but they mean very little pathologically. Yet in every other field of medicine it is well recognized that unless an accurate pathological diagnosis is made, treatment is unlikely to result in relief of the patient's symptoms.

45

General Examination

POSSIBLE ETIOLOGICAL FACTORS.   I venture to say that virtually never does a clinician examine the knee as a possible source of pain in the foot or ankle, yet a malfunctioning superior tibiofibular joint can give rise to acute pain in the lateral aspect of the ankle and foot (see pages 78–79).

One does not often see an examiner feeling the pulses of the legs of a patient with the simple complaint of foot pain, at least initially; and it is only recently that clinicians have become aware of entrapment syndromes in the lower extremity which give rise to pain in the foot.

Moreover, clinicians rarely understand the importance of the appreciation of the relative sufficiency or insufficiency of the Achilles tendons. Achilles tendon insufficiency is associated with an accentuation of the drop of the forefoot at rest, resulting, in the course of time, in myostatic contractures of the intrinsic muscles of the foot and shortening of the plantar fascia, which in turn results in impairment of the function of the joints of the foot. This condition, which is discussed at greater lengths in Chapter 6, is often associated with taut iliotibial bands and chronic sacroiliac or lumbosacral joint problems, part of the treatment of which must be attention to the condition of the feet.

In considering the living foot, as in consideration of any part of the musculoskeletal system, it is my experience that, in the absence of frank disease, musculoskeletal pain symptoms most commonly arise from a condition, which I call "joint dysfunction," that results from a loss of joint play in synovial joints. At least joint dysfunction plays a part in the etiological complex of almost all pain in the foot. In every live synovial joint, as in every mechanical thing that is made to move, there is a built-in factor of joint play. In the human being the range of movement of joint play at each synovial joint is specific to that joint, though there may be an individual variation in the extent of each movement. Normal joint-play movements cannot be performed by muscle action, and if they are lost, muscles cannot perform the normal voluntary movements of the joint, for functional joint movement is dependent upon the presence of normal joint play. Clinical examination, therefore, is incomplete unless a diligent search is made for the presence of normal joint play in all of the synovial joints in the foot.

General Physical Examination. TEMPERATURE AND PULSE. The patient's temperature and pulse should be taken before any examination of the painful part is undertaken. This may be a trite observation, but these two simple examining procedures are too often overlooked. This is just as important in a patient with foot pain as it is in a patient with pain anywhere else in the musculo-skeletal system.

Besides general patient assessment there are, of course, special reasons for assessing the pulses in relation to the search for a cause of foot pain. Vascular diseases, which are discussed in Chapter 5, are a common cause of foot pain, and special investigations may have to be undertaken in such cases. These include oscillometry, the use of ice water producing contralateral reflex vasospasm or hot water not producing distant reflex vasodilation — the Landis-Gibbon test — and the use of differential heating in a constant-temperature room. However, these tests lie in the province of the specialist in peripheral vascular diseases.

INSPECTION.   Any painful part of the musculoskeletal system should be inspected before it is palpated or moved. The color of the skin and the presence or absence of swelling should be noted. Any alteration of muscle contour or noticeable muscle atrophy is important. In the foot, the bulge of the extensor brevis digitorum muscle is often found to be absent when a patient is suffering from prolapse of a low lumbar disc, for instance. The appearance of the normal foot should always be compared with that of the painful foot.

PALPATION.   Before the foot is moved at all, it should be palpated at rest. At this time differences of local skin temperature, the presence of fluctuation in any part of it, the consistency of the joint capsules and of the supporting and mobilizing muscles, both extrinsic and intrinsic, their tendons and tendon sheaths must be noted. At this point I would reiterate the importance of examining the superior tibiofibular joint in the complete examination of the patient with foot pain.

The discrete ligaments of the ankle and foot must be examined by palpation individually because of the fact that ligaments are never tender unless they are torn or ruptured or unless there is some pathological condition within the joint which they support. In the foot there is one discrete ligament of the subtalar joint palpable through the sinus tarsi which must not be overlooked on examination.

Normal capsules of synovial joints cannot be appreciated on palpation, and if a capsule can be felt, there is some serious pathological condition present.

EXAMINATION OF MOVEMENTS IN THE VOLUNTARY RANGE. In the presence of signs of active inflammation within a joint, which can be detected by the examination procedures described up to this point, it is then unnecessary to examine joint movement at all.

In the absence of signs of active inflammation in the foot, movements of the joints of the foot in their voluntary range should be noted as they are performed actively by the patient and then should be checked by passive examination. The degrees of movement in each normal range of movement should be noted in the unaffected foot, and the loss of movement in the affected foot should be noted as a baseline from which improvement or deterioration can be checked. The leg lengths should be measured, since inequality of leg length may cause unnatural stresses of weight bearing on an otherwise normal foot and may result in joint dysfunction from relatively innocuous unguarded movements. It may also be the cause of changes of traumatic osteoarthritis or strain of supporting ligaments of the joints at the ankle or in the foot from constant, repetitive strain from otherwise normal function. At this point the sufficiency of the Achilles tendons should be noted (see page 200).

Study of the gait should be undertaken, and deviation of normal functioning of the foot as described in Chapter 3 should be noted. Correction of the gait may be an integral part of the overall treatment of the painful foot condition.

Study of the patient's footwear may also provide clues to mechanical problems of the feet. The shoes should be examined outside for abnormal wear patterns and inside for worn linings and other abnormal ridges or projecting nails.

MUSCLE EXAMINATION. It is almost impossible to examine the function of the intrinsic muscles of the foot because of their alienation from disuse, but examination of the extrinsic muscles of the foot together with their tendons and tendon sheaths must be undertaken. A manual muscle test is often an important part of the clinical examination, providing a baseline from which improvement or deterioration of a pathological condition may be assessed. Electromyography is of value only when some interruption of the neuromuscular mechanism or some muscle disease is present. Muscle volume and power should always be compared with that on the unaffected side.

X-ray Examination. Little heed is taken of the fact that, except in the case of fractures, it probably takes months, if not years, before gross radiographic changes become apparent; that symptoms of a few weeks or even months are unlikely to be arising from the radiographic changes which probably preceded them by a considerable period of time; and that if the symptoms are completely relieved by proper treatment, as they well may be, the radiographic appearance of the foot appears unaltered. Thus, radiographic changes may precede and succeed symptoms without alteration. For example, a patient may have rheumatoid arthritis with gross rheumatoid changes in the feet, but the pain in the feet may have nothing to do with the rheumatoid process at all.

The habit of looking at x-ray films of the foot before undertaking the clinical examination is depreciated. Obvious radiographic changes in the bones and joints of the foot do not necessarily mean that these are the causes of the patient's symptoms. X-rays, for the most part, should be used to confirm a clinical diagnosis and not to make it. There are no characteristic radiographic changes in joints to suggest the diagnosis of joint dysfunction, and joint dysfunction may be present and giving rise to symptoms in the absence or presence of any radiographic changes.

One should not even rely on x-rays to diagnose fractures; in the foot there are bones — that is, the calcaneus, the talus, and neck of the metatarsal bones — in which a fracture may not be shown by x-ray until 10 days or more have passed following injury.

Sometimes special x-ray techniques are needed before an accurate diagnosis can be arrived at. Stress radiographs may have to be taken to determine the integrity of the supporting ligaments, especially at the mortise joint. Stereoscopic films may help to locate loose bodies within a joint. Planigrams may have to be undertaken to reveal early bone destruction which is otherwise undetectable because not enough bone has been destroyed to be visible on routine films.

When investigating the possibility that foot pain may be due to vascular disease, the special x-ray techniques of arteriography and venography may have to be used.

Laboratory Procedures. Certain laboratory tests may be required before an accurate diagnosis of the cause of foot pain can be arrived at. A complete blood count and erythrocyte sedimentation rate should be almost routine. A determination of the serum uric acid may lead to the diagnosis of gout. An estimation of the albumin-globulin ratio and the performance of the usual complement-fixation, flocculation, and agglutination tests may be necessary before conditions such as rheumatoid arthritis, brucellosis, or syphilis, for instance, can be diagnosed or ruled out. A hematological study for lupus erythematosus may be necessary, and such nonspecific determinations as the C-reactive protein, in conjunction with other laboratory studies, may be useful. Certainly, serial determinations of the antistreptolysin-O titer may be essential in revealing or following the activity of rheumatic fever. The heterophil antibody may reveal infectious mononucleosis to be the underlying problem. Sickle-cell preparations in a Negro may give the clue to the correct diagnosis. Parasitic ova may have to be sought for in the stools. Urinalysis, urine culture, and such procedures as throat culture and blood cultures may have to be done. Skin tests may also be necessary.

A painful joint may have to be aspirated for diagnostic purposes. The cellular content of synovial fluid may give a clue to the pathological condition within the joint, and the synovial fluid may have to be cultured to determine the organism causing infection and its sensitivity to antibiotics. There are times when synovial biopsy is essential to arrive at the correct diagnosis of the cause of foot pain.

Other Procedures. When investigating the possibility that foot pain may be due to primary pathology in the central or peripheral nervous system, it may be necessary to do not only a complete neurological examination but also an analysis of the cerebrospinal fluid. In such cases the various electrodiagnostic testing procedures — electromyography, nerve conduction studies, chronaxie determinations, or even the reaction of degeneration test — may have to be undertaken.

Examination of Movements of Joint Play

While it is true that many of the foregoing auxiliary diagnostic procedures are often unnecessary and even redundant in arriving at the correct diagnosis of the cause of foot pain, they have been discussed in this order to reemphasize the fact that joint dysfunction is but an additional diagnostic conclusion to be arrived at in assessing the problem of foot pain. By the same token, it should not be forgotten, and it is also pertinent to differential diagnosis, that joint dysfunction is one of the commonest causes of pain in the feet. Evidence of joint dysfunction is therefore sought early, in the absence of any clinical signs to suggest more serious pathological causes of pain.

Causes of Joint Dysfunction. The etiological factors that cause a loss of joint play are: (1) intrinsic trauma, which usually means the imposition of an unguarded movement at a joint during the performance of a normal functional movement; (2) immobilization; (3) disuse; (4) aging; and (5) the resolution of some more serious injury or disease.

In the human foot, immobilization and disuse are common features of twentieth-century living, the former being caused by the shape and style of shoes dictated by fashion and shoe manufacturers, and the latter being caused by laziness in the age of the automobile.

Rules for Joint-Play Examination. To examine for joint-play movements in the joints of the foot, the patient must be recumbent; only in this position does the examiner have perfect control of the examining movements that he is performing. The techniques of eliciting joint play must be adhered to. It must be remembered that joint-play movements, for the most part, are small in range, and therefore their performance requires accuracy and precision. In addition, there are certain rules of examining technique which must be followed when using manipulative maneuvers.

1. The patient must be relaxed, and each aspect of the joint being examined must be supported and protected from unguarded painful movement which may otherwise occur in the course of the examination. Unguarded movements of painful joints produce pain which puts the supporting muscles into spasm and prevents the performance of the examining movements for joint play.

2. The examiner must be relaxed, and at no time must his examining grip be painful to the patient; the grip must be firm and protective, but not restrictive.

3. One joint must be examined at a time; this is stressed in the topographical portion of this chapter.

4. One movement at each joint is examined at a time.

5. In the performance of any one movement, one articular surface of the joint being examined is moved on the other articular surface which is stabilized. Thus, there should always be one mobilizing force and one stabilizing force exerted when a joint is being examined.

6. The extent of normal joint play can usually be ascertained by examining the same joint in the unaffected foot.

7. No forceful movement must ever be used, and no abnormal movement must ever be used.

8. An examining movement must be stopped at any point at which pain is elicited. This is in contradistinction to rule 8 in the rules concerning therapeutic techniques using manipulative maneuvers described in Chapter 8.

9. In the presence of obvious clinical signs of joint (or bone) inflammation or disease, no examining movements need be or should be taken.

EXCEPTIONS TO RULES OF JOINT-PLAY EXAMINATION. In the following section, which describes the topographical examination of the joints of the foot, it will be noted that rules 3 and 4 may be broken. For instance, in examining for long axis extension of the subtalar joint, the movement of long axis extension of the mortise joint is also achieved. Also, in performing the other movements of joint play in the the subtalar joint (i.e., talar rock and the lateral and medial tilt movements of the calcaneus on the talus), it will be noted that these movements can be elicited only with the joint in long axis extension. However, in eliciting these joint-play movements in the subtalar joint, the rules are deliberately broken. The key word in the foregoing sentence is *deliberately.* The only time that the user of manipulative techniques may break these rules is when he knowingly does it for a specific technical reason. If the rule is broken unknowingly, damage may be inflicted on the joint being examined. If the rules are broken unknowingly when a therapeutic manipulation is being performed, severe injury may be inflicted upon the joint being treated, and the novice will blame the procedure rather than his lack of knowledge of the technique for the increased joint symptoms or the failure of the treatment to bring relief to his patient.

Techniques of Joint-Play Examination

We must next consider the techniques used for examination of the joints of the feet for joint play and learn the extent of the normal range of joint play at the various synovial joints of the toes, the foot, and the ankle and at the superior tibiofibular joint of the knee, for it is only when one knows the extent of normal that one can detect its loss — that is, what is abnormal.

The Metatarsophalangeal and Interphalangeal Joints

The range of joint play in the metatarsophalangeal joints and the interphalangeal joints is the same, though the extent of each movement is different and the facility with which they may be performed is less because of the anatomical structure of the soft parts of the foot. Fortunately, in clinical practice one is usually limited to examining the metatarsophalangeal joints, since the phalangeal joints of the toes seldom are involved in pain-producing dysfunction.

The metatarsophalangeal joint of the big toe is used to illustrate the range of joint-play movement in all these joints. The movements of joint play at this joint are: (1) long axis extension, (2) anteroposterior tilt, (3) side tilt medially and laterally, and (4) rotation.

LONG AXIS EXTENSION.   The examiner holds the head of the metatarsal bone between the thumb and the index finger of his right hand and grasps the base of the proximal phalanx between the thumb and index finger of his left hand, the thumb of the left hand being placed on the dorsal aspect of the base of the proximal phalanx and the left index finger being placed on its plantar aspect. He then pulls the proximal phalanx away from

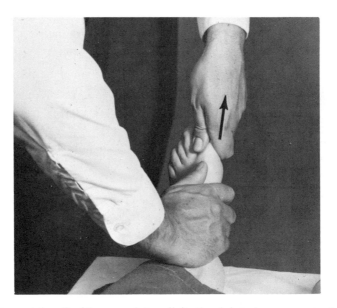

FIGURE 4-1. Position used to elicit the joint-play movement of long axis extension at the metatarsophalangeal joint of the big toe. Note the golf-club grip by the examiner's left hand and stabilization of the head of the metatarsal by his right hand. Arrow shows direction of pull.

the head of the metatarsal bone in the direction of the long axis of the toe. The position adopted to perform this movement is shown in Figure 4-1.

ANTEROPOSTERIOR TILT. The examiner maintains the grip upon the head of the metatarsal bone with his right hand and places the tip of his left thumb just distal to the base of the proximal phalanx dorsally and the tip of his left index finger just distal to the base of the phalanx on its plantar surface. Using the left thumb and the left index finger alternately as a fulcrum, the examiner tilts the base of the subject's phalanx alternately backward and forward, opening either the dorsal or the plantar aspect of the joint. The posterior phase of this joint-play movement, as

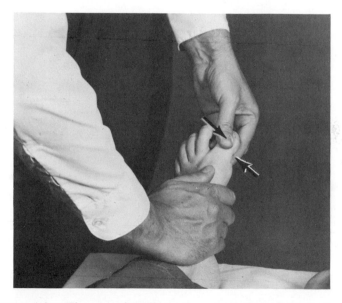

FIGURE 4-2. The posterior tilt at the completion of the posterior phase of the anteroposterior tilt at the first metatarsophalangeal joint. Note the examiner's left index finger being used as a pivot (*lower arrow*) on the plantar aspect of the proximal phalanx, while the thumb presses forward (*upper arrow*) over it.

well as the position adopted to elicit it, is shown in Figure 4-2.
There is actually a mobilizing force in both finger and thumb in
each movement.

SIDE TILT MEDIALLY AND LATERALLY.   The examiner maintains his grip on the head of the metatarsal bone with his right
hand. He places the tip of his left thumb deep in the web between
the first and second toes and the tip of the left index finger
medially just distal to the base of the proximal phalanx. Using
the thumb as a pivot, the metatarsophalangeal joint is tilted
open on its medial aspect by exerting pressure through the tip
of the left index finger, using the tip of the left thumb as a fulcrum.

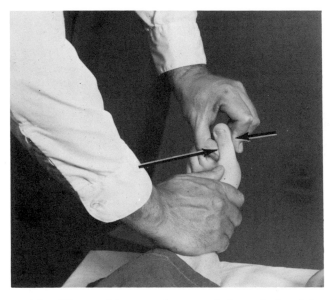

FIGURE 4-3. The position at the completion of the joint-play
movement of side tilt laterally, opening up the medial aspect of the
first metatarsophalangeal joint. Note that the examiner's left thumb
is being used as a pivot, while the index finger tilts the base of the
phalanx laterally on the metatarsal bone. The forces of the thumb
and index finger are reversed to achieve the side tilt medially to
open up the lateral aspect of the joint.

Then, using the tip of the index finger as a pivot, the metatarsophalangeal joint is tilted open laterally by exerting pressure through the thumb. Figure 4-3 illustrates the position at the completion of the medial phase of the joint-play movement of side tilt as well as the position adopted to elicit this movement. There is actually a mobilizing force in both finger and thumb in each movement.

ROTATION.   The examiner maintains his grip on the head of the metatarsal bone with his right hand. The interphalangeal joint of the big toe is flexed. The examiner then grasps the proximal phalanx with his left thumb and index and middle fingers, and hooks the distal phalanx of his fourth and fifth fingers on the lateral aspect of the subject's distal flexed phalanx. The examiner rotates the proximal phalanx on the metatarsal head alternately clockwise and counterclockwise in its long axis. The position adopted to elicit this movement is shown in Figure 4-4.

The joint-play movements of the other metatarsophalangeal joints and the interphalangeal joints are elicited in the same way, only the degree of normal movement being different.

The Distal Intermetatarsal Joints.   The movements of joint play between the heads of each metatarsal bone are: (1) anteroposterior glide and (2) rotation. Of course the joints between these bones are not true synovial joints anatomically, but functionally the movement between them may be impaired; if so, dysfunction occurs, and the symptoms of pain are produced just as though they were synovial joints. The stationary axis is the second metatarsal bone.

ANTEROPOSTERIOR GLIDE.   With the subject in the recumbent position, the examiner sits at the end of the couch, facing the

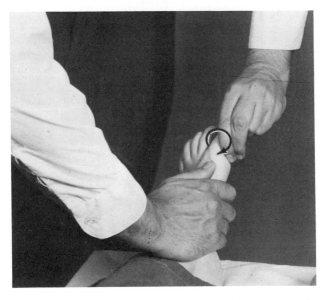

FIGURE 4-4. Rotation of the base of the phalanx on the head of the metatarsal bone of the big toe. The model's distal phalanx is flexed, and the distal phalanges of the examiner's fourth and fifth fingers are on its lateral aspect. Leverage is thus achieved that ensures that rotation is in the long axis of the proximal phalanx.

plantar aspect of the subject's foot. (The left foot is used for illustration.) The examiner grasps the neck of the second metatarsal bone, his right thumb being on the plantar aspect and his fingers on the dorsal aspect of it. He grasps the metatarsal bone of the first toe in a similar manner with his left hand. The second metatarsal bone is stabilized, and the head of the first metatarsal bone is moved upward and downward upon it. The reader should remember that the words *upward* and *downward* are used in an anatomical sense but the movement of the heads of the metatarsal bones is positionally *forward* and *backward*.

The role of the examiner's hands is then reversed. He grasps the second metatarsal bone with his left hand and with his right (mobilizing) hand moves the head of the third metatarsal bone upward and downward upon it. He then stabilizes the third metatarsal bone with his left hand and with his right hand moves the head of the fourth metatarsal bone upward and downward upon it. Finally, the fourth metatarsal bone is stabilized with the examiner's left hand and the head of the fifth metatarsal bone is moved upward and downward upon it. The movement of the head of the fifth metatarsal bone upon the head of the fourth is shown in Figure 4-5.

ROTATION. The examiner stabilizes the head of the second metatarsal bone in the same way that has been described above in the examination to elicit the joint-play movement of antero-posterior glide. He then grasps the neck of the first metatarsal bone between his left thumb and index finger, which are now

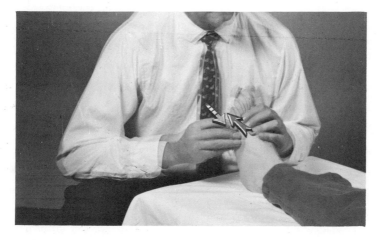

FIGURE 4-5. The joint-play movement of anteroposterior glide of the head of the fifth metatarsal bone on the head of the fourth. The double exposure illustrates the range of the (posterior) phase of the joint-play movement. (It must be remembered that the second metatarsal bone is the axis in the foot so that the head of the fifth metatarsal bone moves about the head of the fourth, the head of the fourth moves about the head of the third, the head of the third moves about the head of the second, and the head of the first moves about the head of the second.)

placed at right angles to the long axis of the metatarsal bone. With a shoulder swing, he rotates the head of the first metatarsal bone in the long axis of its shaft clockwise and counterclockwise upon the head of the second metatarsal bone.

The role of the examiner's hands is then reversed, his left hand now stabilizing the second metatarsal bone. The neck of the third metatarsal bone is grasped between the examiner's right thumb and index finger, placed at right angles to its long axis, and with a shoulder swing he rotates it clockwise and counter-clockwise on the stabilized head of the second metatarsal bone. The examiner then stabilizes the third metatarsal bone with his left hand and with his right hand rotates the head of the fourth metatarsal bone on the head of the third. The examiner finally stabilizes the fourth metatarsal bone and rotates the head of the fifth metatarsal bone on the head of the fourth. Figure 4-6 illustrates the position adopted to produce this last movement, the double exposure showing the extent of the movement.

The Tarsometatarsal Joints.   The movements of the tarsomet-atarsal joints are all in the involuntary range. There are also facets between the bases of the metatarsal bones which are, in fact, part of the synovial joints. Joint-play movements at the tarsometatarsal joints and proximal intermetatarsal joints are: (1) anteroposterior glide and (2) rotation.

ANTEROPOSTERIOR GLIDE.   The distal tarsal bones are grasped in relation to the base of the metatarsal bones. Using the right foot for illustration, the bases of the metatarsal bones are grasped over their dorsal aspect by the examiner's right hand, while his left hand stabilizes the distal tarsal bones. His mobiliz-ing right hand alternately thrusts upward and downward, per-forming an anteroposterior glide movement (superoinferior in

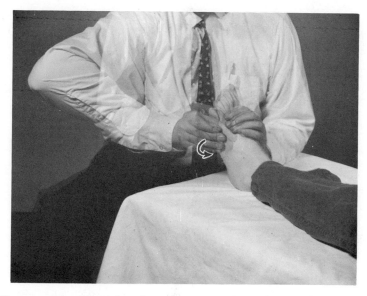

FIGURE 4-6. The joint-play movement of rotation of the head of the fifth metatarsal bone on the head of the fourth. The double exposure illustrates the range of the counterclockwise part of the movement. Note that the movement is achieved from the examiner's shoulder.

direction) between the bases of the metatarsal bones and the adjacent tarsal bones. Figure 4-7 illustrates this movement. The base of the fifth metatarsal bone can be moved independently on the cuboid bone to elicit the anteroposterior glide specific to this joint.

ROTATION. There is a different degree of rotation of the bases of the metatarsal bones on their adjacent tarsal bones, and the movement cannot specifically be elicited at each joint but has to be performed at all of the joints at once. Using the right foot for illustration, the examiner faces the lateral aspect of the foot and stabilizes the tarsal bones by grasping them over their dorsal aspect with his left hand. He then cradles the necks of the

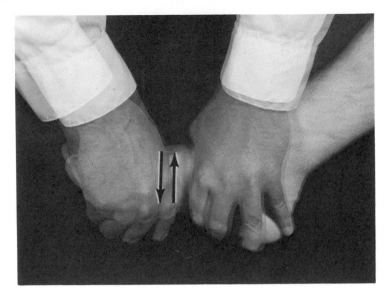

FIGURE 4-7. The position adopted to elicit the joint-play movement of anteroposterior glide at the joints between the bases of the
metatarsal bones and the three cuneiform bones and the cuboid
bone. The double exposure indicates the range of movement downward. The thumb and index finger of the examiner's left (stabilizing) hand must be carefully positioned so that the movement is not
mistakenly elicited at the midtarsal joint—a movement of joint
play illustrated in Figure 4-9.

metatarsal bones between his right thumb, which is placed across
them dorsally, and the four fingers, which are placed across them
on their plantar surface. The examiner then rotates the forefoot
as a whole, first into eversion and then into inversion. This
produces a rotation of the bases of the metatarsal bones upon
the tarsal bones, first clockwise and then counterclockwise.
Figure 4-8 illustrates the position adopted to elicit this movement, the double exposure showing the extent of the clockwise
movement.

The Midtarsal Joints. ANTEROPOSTERIOR GLIDE.   There are
no true voluntary movements of the midtarsal joints, but there

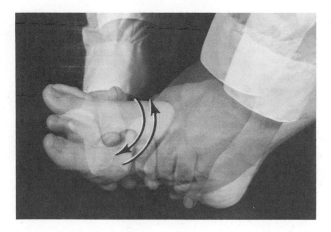

FIGURE 4-8. The position adopted to elicit the movement of rotation of the bases of the metatarsal bones on the distal row of tarsal
bones. The double exposure indicates the clockwise (eversion) part
of this movement; a similar range is obtainable in the counterclockwise (inversion) direction. The thumb and index finger of the examiner's left (stabilizing) hand must be carefully positioned over the
distal tarsal bones so that the joint-play movement is limited to the
tarsometatarsal joints.

is one important involuntary movement upon which the resilience
of the foot to take up the stresses and strains of function largely
depends, that is, an anteroposterior (superoinferior) type of
movement of the distal cuneiform bones on the navicula (scaphoid), and the navicula upon the talus. Using the left foot for
illustration, the examiner stabilizes the navicula and cuboid with
his right hand over the dorsal aspect and grasps the three cuneiform bones with his left hand, moving them upward and downward alternately. He then releases his grip on the navicula by
placing his hand farther back toward the mortise joint and grasps
the talus and calcaneus with his right (mobilizing) hand; he
alternates a dorsal and plantar movement of the navicula and
cuboid on the stabilized talus and calcaneus (Figure 4-9), eliciting an anteroposterior movement. The anteroposterior movements of the navicula on the talus and the cuboid on the cal-

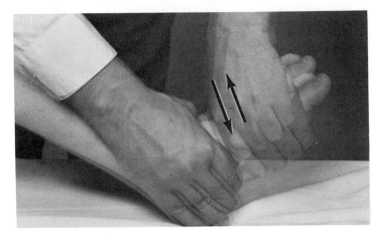

FIGURE 4-9.   The position adopted to elicit the joint-play movement of anteroposterior glide at the midtarsal joint. The double exposure indicates the range of movement downward. The thumb and
index finger of the examiner's right (stabilizing) hand must carefully be positioned to grasp proximally to the articulating surfaces of
the talus and calcaneus. The thumb and index finger of his mobilizing left hand must carefully be positioned over the navicular and
cuboid bones to avoid movement at the wrong joint.

caneus are well elicited by the examining maneuver which is
used to demonstrate long axis extension at the subtalar (subastragaloid) joint (page 73). Figure 4-16 shows radiographically the extent to which the navicula and the cuboid move.

The Intertarsal Joints. FORWARD AND BACKWARD SHIFTS.
There is, of course, a range of movement (superoinferior in
direction) between each tarsal bone. This cannot be appreciated
clinically on examination unless there has been a traumatic subluxation of one of the bones upon another. The subluxation is
usually upward, and there is a clinical sign of pain on pressing
the affected bone downward on examination. The range of the
specific involuntary movement probably consists of each bone's
moving slightly upward and downward upon its neighbor.

The Mortise Joint.   The mortise joint is made up of the lower tibial condyle and the tibial and fibular malleoli, which constitute one joint aspect, and the superior aspect of the talus (astragalus). There are but two movements of joint play at this joint: (1) long axis extension and (2) anteroposterior glide.

LONG AXIS EXTENSION.   The examiner sits on the couch with his back to the subject, who is lying supine with his hip abducted and flexed to not less than 90 degrees and whose knee is also flexed to a right angle. Using the right foot for illustration, the examiner grasps the lower leg around the ankle, the left thenar web being placed posteriorly to the Achilles tendon and the right thenar web being placed over the dorsum of the foot as close to the ankle as possible. The examiner then leans backward on the subject's thigh while he pushes the foot away from him in the long axis of the lower leg, maintaining the foot at a right angle to it. Figure 4-10 illustrates the position adopted for the examining maneuver, and the double exposure shows the extent of the movement of long axis extension.

ANTEROPOSTERIOR GLIDE.   With the subject recumbent and the hip, knee, and ankle all at 90-degree angles, the examiner grasps the subject's lower leg around the ankle just above the malleoli with his left hand; he grasps the dorsum of the foot with the right hand, which will stabilize it during the performance of this movement. The mobilizing left hand then pulls forward and pushes backward alternately, thereby moving the mortise forward and backward upon the immobile superior talar facet. Figure 4-11 shows the position adopted for eliciting this movement.

The Subtalar (Subastragaloid) Joint.   Anatomy texts describe this joint simply as the joint between the talus and the calcaneus

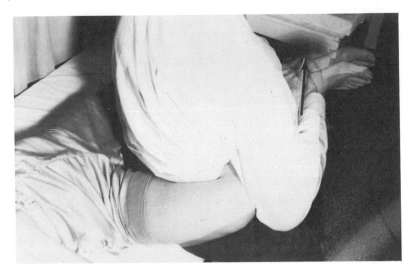

FIGURE 4-10. The position adopted to elicit the joint-play movement of long axis extension at the mortise joint. Note that the hip, knee, and ankle are held at right angles. The examiner thrusts forward in the long axis of the tibia, exerting countertraction by leaning backward against the posterior aspect of the model's thigh. Note that the thrust of the examiner's hands is through the web between his thumbs and index fingers, and there is no true grip on the sides of the model's foot. The double exposure illustrates the extent of the joint-play movement of long axis extension.

whose range of movement is that of inversion and eversion at the ankle. In fact, the function of this joint is far from simple; its most important movement, which is seldom described, is a rocking movement of the talus upon the calcaneus which is entirely independent of voluntary muscle action. It is this movement that takes up all the stresses and strains of stubbing the toes and that spares the ankle from gross trauma, both at toe-off and at heel strike, in the normal function of walking and when abnormal stresses that tend to twist the ankle to a great extent are inflicted at the ankle joint. If it were not for this involuntary rocking motion at the subtalar joint, fracture dislocations around the ankle would be commonplace.

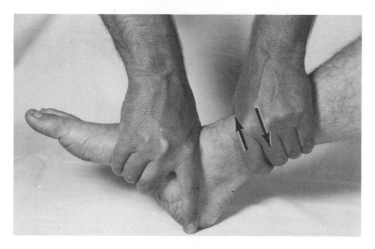

FIGURE 4-11. The position adopted to elicit the anteroposterior glide of the articulating surfaces of the tibia and fibula on the talus. The examiner's right hand is the mobilizing hand. Note that the foot is held at right angles to the lower leg by the examiner's right (stabilizing) hand; the model's knee and hip are flexed.

DIFFERENTIATION OF MOVEMENT FROM THE MORTISE JOINT. The importance of clinical differentiation of mortise joint pain from subtalar joint pain cannot be too highly stressed. This differentiation is quite easily achieved, however. With the subject recumbent and the hip, knee, and ankle all at right angles, the examiner grasps the lower leg some 6 inches above the malleoli with his left hand and supports the sole of the foot with his right hand. The subject's foot is now resting upon the posteroinferior angle of the calcaneus, and the examiner rocks the foot on it by pushing upward and downward on the tibia, thereby producing plantar flexion and dorsiflexion of the foot at the mortise joint. If these movements are full, free, and painless, there is obviously no pathological condition in this joint. The position adopted for these examining maneuvers and the normal range of voluntary movement at the mortise joint are shown in Figure 4-12.

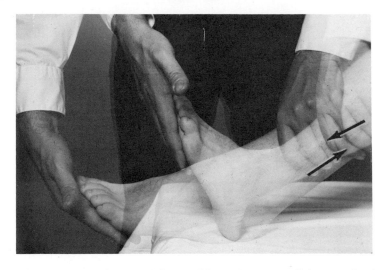

FIGURE 4-12.   The examining position adopted to elicit pure dorsiflexion and plantar flexion at the mortise joint. The double exposure illustrates the extent of this voluntary movement. The examiner's left hand elicits the movement by rocking the foot on the
posteroinferior angle of the calcaneus. His right hand simply maintains the sole of the foot in its unchanging plane.

TALAR ROCK.   To examine for the normal rocking movement
at the subtalar joint, instead of stopping the plantar-flexion movement at its limit, the examiner now pushes through the limit of
this movement, thereby producing the rock of the talus on the calcaneus. This movement is not one of hyper–plantar flexion which,
if performed, simply puts an abnormal stretch upon the anterior
transverse ligament of the ankle joint and produces pain; such
pain simply indicates that an abnormal movement is being performed at the mortise joint. The talar rock is produced as the
thrust of the examiner's hand down the tibia is resisted by friction
where the calcaneus is resting on the couch. This friction force
is sufficient to stabilize the calcaneus while the talus rocks forward upon it. The range of the talar rock beyond full plantar
flexion at the mortise joint is shown in Figure 4-13. Pain on

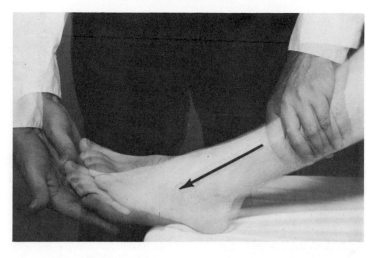

FIGURE 4-13. The additional movement of apparent plantar flexion that is obtained when the joint-play talar rock is brought into
play. The examiner thrusts down the long axis of the tibia with his
left hand (*arrow*) through the limit of plantar flexion, which is illustrated in Figure 4-12. The double exposure shows how the foot slips
forward slightly on the couch, indicating that this is not forced
plantar flexion. The examiner's right hand simply guides the foot
in an unchanging plane.

the performance of this movement indicates some pathological
condition giving rise to pain in the subtalar joint. Figure 4-14
is a lateral radiographic view of a normal ankle, and the appearance of the subtalar joint should be noted and compared with
its appearance when the movements of joint play are being elicited
(see Figs. 4-19 and 4-20).

The stress of inversion or eversion of the foot may be added
while performing this movement if the examiner keeps the sole
of the foot in the horizontal plane with his supporting hand and
exerts a lateral or medial thrust upon the subject's lower leg,
using his left forearm, during the performance of this movement.
Further clinical evidence of pathology in the subtalar joint is
obtained by noting that maximum tenderness is elicited on pal-

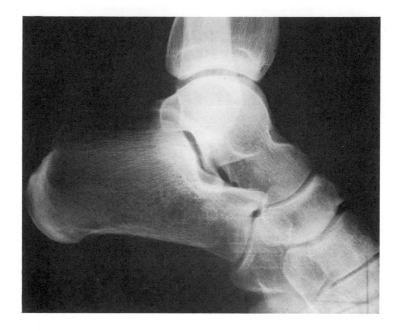

FIGURE 4-14.   A lateral radiographic view of a normal ankle joint.
The appearance of the subtalar (subastragaloid) joint should be
kept in mind when studying the illustrations of joint-play movement at this important joint.

pating through the sinus tarsi and that localized swelling is
situated in relationship to this area, rather than tenderness and
swelling being in relationship to the fibular malleolus and the
fibular collateral ligament.

The joint-play movements at the subtalar joint are: (1) long
axis extension, (2) rock of talus on calcaneus, (3) side tilt
medially, and (4) side tilt laterally.

LONG AXIS EXTENSION.   The examiner adopts the examining
position that has already been described for eliciting the joint-
play movement of long axis extension at the mortise joint. Long
axis extension at the subtalar joint cannot be performed without

exerting long axis extension at the mortise joint. In eliciting this movement, then, one deliberately breaks one of the cardinal rules of manipulative technique in that two movements are performed at the same time. Figure 4-15 illustrates the position adopted for eliciting the movement of long axis extension, the double exposure indicating the extent of the movement elicited. The extent of the movement illustrated, of course, is the summation of long axis extension at the mortise joint and at the subtalar joint.

Figure 4-16 is a lateral radiographic view of a normal ankle at the completion of the joint-play movement of long axis extension at the subtalar joint. Clearly, long axis extension cannot be elicited at this joint without exerting long axis extension

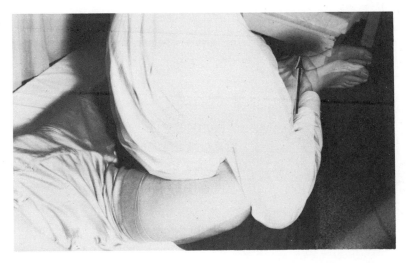

FIGURE 4-15. The position adopted to elicit the joint-play movement of long axis extension at the subtalar joint is exactly the same as that in Figure 4-10, which illustrates long axis extension at the mortise joint. (The technique used to elicit movement is described in caption to Figure 4-10.) The extent of the range of this movement is, of course, a summation of long axis extension at both the mortise and the subtalar joints.

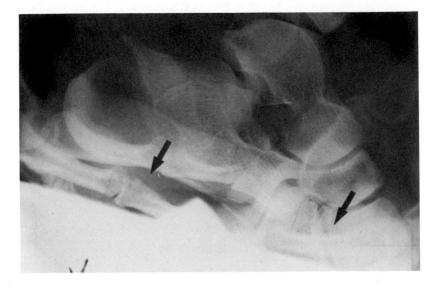

FIGURE 4-16. The subtalar (subastragaloid) joint at the completion of the joint-play movement of long axis extension. The arrows
indicate the direction of the thrusts of the examiner's hands.

at the mortise joint also. The extent of this movement at the
mortise joint is just apparent.

It is interesting to note the joint-play movements of the cuboid
on the calcaneus and of the navicula on the talus which are
elicited during the performance of long axis extension at the
subtalar joint. It is analogous to an anteroposterior glide, the
posterior phase of which occurs on the rebound when the examining stress is released. These movements were alluded to previously in the discussion of the joint play at the midtarsal joint
(see page 64).

ROCK OF TALUS ON CALCANEUS.   The previous description
of the talar rock was limited to its examination while the foot

and ankle are in function. The examination for this specific rocking movement is now described. The position adopted by the examiner is the same as that used for eliciting the movement of long axis extension. In reproducing the joint-play movement of the talar rock, it is again necessary to perform two joint-play movements at the same time because the talar rock cannot be performed passively unless the joint is in the position of long axis extension.

Holding the foot and leg with the subtalar and mortise joints in the position of the limit of long axis extension, the examiner now pushes upward and forward with the hand which is behind the Achilles tendon, thereby rocking the calcaneus forward on

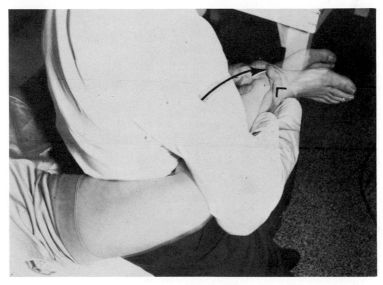

FIGURE 4-17. The extent of the forward movement of the calcaneus on the talus, which is the posterior phase of the talar rock. Note that movement is elicited while full long axis extension at the mortise and subtalar joints is maintained. The examiner's left hand acts as the mobilizer (*arrow*), pressure being exerted on the posterior aspect of the calcaneus by the web between the thumb and index finger.

the talus (Fig. 4-17). Then the examiner pushes backward and downward with the hand that is on the anterodorsal aspect of the foot to produce the posterior rock of the calcaneus on the talus (Fig. 4-18). Figures 4-19 and 4-20 are x-rays taken at the completion of the forward and backward phases of the talar rock. Figure 4-19 corresponds to the foot illustrated in Figure 4-17; Figure 4-20 corresponds to the foot in Figure 4-18.

These movements have nothing to do with the movements of plantar flexion and dorsiflexion, which must be studiously avoided. This rocking movement of the subtalar joint is best appreciated by comparing the feeling of it with that of the dorsiflexion and plantar-flexion movements that take place at the mortise joint.

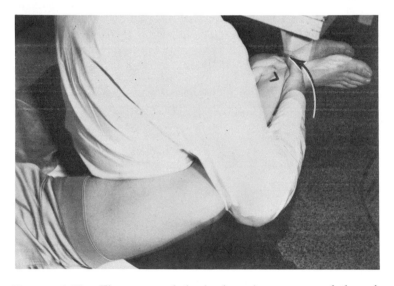

FIGURE 4-18. The extent of the backward movement of the calcaneus on the talus, which is the anterior phase of the talar rock. Note that movement is elicited while full long axis extension at the mortise and subtalar joints is maintained. The examiner's right (mobilizing) hand is exerting pressure indirectly on the anterior aspect of the calcaneus through the other tarsal bones by the web between the thumb and index finger.

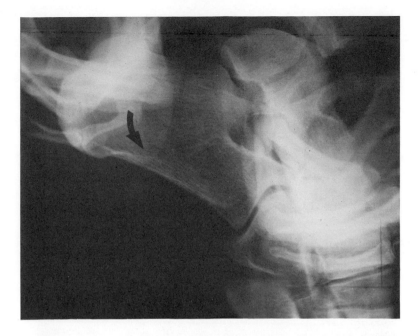

FIGURE 4-19. The subtalar joint at the completion of the posterior phase of the talar rock. The arrow indicates the direction of the thrust of the examiner's hand over the posterior aspect of the calcaneus.

SIDE TILT MEDIALLY. Again, the position adopted to elicit this movement is the same as that described for the previous movements, and again one of the rules of manipulation technique is deliberately broken, as more than one movement is performed at a time. The tilting movement, both medially and laterally, can only be achieved when the joint is at the limit of long axis extension. So, to elicit the movement of side tilt medially, first long axis extension is performed, as illustrated in Figure 4-15. When long axis extension is achieved, the examiner's thumbs, which are placed on the medial aspect of the calcaneus, thrust laterally upon the calcaneus, tilting the subtalar joint open on its

medial aspect. This movement is that of a pure tilt of the calcaneus upon the talus and is not simple eversion of the foot at
the subtalar joint. The extent of this movement is shown in
Figure 4-21.

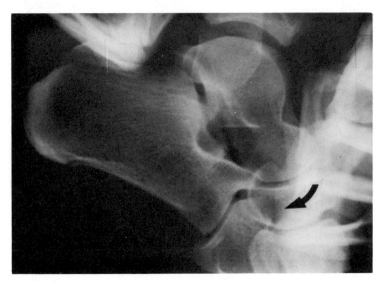

FIGURE 4-20.   The subtalar joint at the completion of the anterior
phase of the talar rock. The arrow indicates the direction of the
thrust of the examiner's hand indirectly through the other tarsal
bones over the anterior aspect of the calcaneus. This movement corresponds with that illustrated in Figure 4-18.

SIDE TILT LATERALLY.   This movement is elicited in exactly
the same way as the movement of the side tilt medially, but
instead of producing the tilting thrust through the thumbs on the
medial aspect of the calcaneus, the tilting thrust is imparted
through the fingers which are placed over the lateral aspect of
the calcaneus. Figure 4-22 shows the extent of this movement.

The Superior Tibiofibular Joint.   The only movement of joint
play at this joint is the anteroposterior glide.

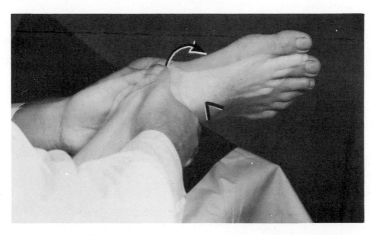

FIGURE 4-21. The movement of side tilt medially of the calcaneus upon the talus, which tilts open the subtalar joint on its
medial aspect. Note that movement is elicited while full long axis
extension at the mortise and subtalar joints is maintained. The
thrusting force (*arrow*) is through the examiner's thumbs on the
medial aspect of the calcaneus. His fingers laterally are used as a
pivot. The double exposure illustrates the extent of the movement.

If the joint play of the superior tibiofibular joint is lost and
there is pain from dysfunction of it, the patient may complain
of pain in the knee, but most often he complains of pain in the
ankle. This is understandable when one realizes that this joint
does not really play any part in the function of the knee joint
proper. However, minor impairment of movement in it will
produce greatly magnified impairment of movement of the talofibular part of the mortise joint mechanically because of the long
lever arm. Pain will also be felt in the foot because of a series
of pathophysiological events.

The range of the joint-play movement varies with the degree
of knee flexion and is absent with the knee in full extension. It
is maximal with the knee in midflexion and is demonstrated in
this position.

The examiner sits on the subject's foot with the knee in the

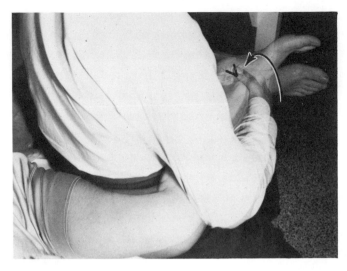

FIGURE 4-22.   The movement of side tilt laterally of the calcaneus upon the talus, which opens up the joint on its lateral aspect. Note that movement is elicited while full long axis extension at the mortise and subtalar joints is maintained. The thrusting force is through the fingers of both hands of the examiner on the lateral aspect of the calcaneus; medially the thumbs are used as pivots. The double exposure illustrates the extent of the movement.

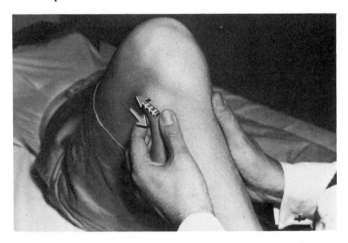

FIGURE 4-23. The position adopted to elicit the anteroposterior movement at the right superior tibiofibular joint. The exposure is made at the limit of the anterior phase of the movement. The examiner's right hand stabilizes the tibia, while his left hand mobilizes the head of the fibula.

required angle of flexion. The head of the fibula is grasped between the thumb anteriorly and the tips of the index and middle fingers posteriorly, and the fingers and thumb then push forward and backward alternately. Figure 4-23 shows the examining position at the completion of the anterior phase of the movement.

Thermography

Thermography is a relatively new diagnostic aid especially useful in determining vascular integrity, and therefore of use in diagnosing the presence of arterial disease. Figure 4-24 shows thermograms of a pair of feet in which arterial insufficiency was suspected in the right foot. Thermography, however, clearly demonstrates a cold spot at the end of the big toe on the left foot and generalized arterial deficiency in the whole foot. Thermography can also be used in the diagnosis of joint diseases and neoplasms, but with less specificity.

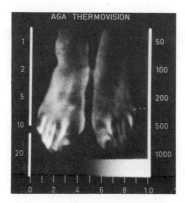

FIGURE 4-24.   Thermogram showing deficient circulation (indicated by increased darkness). Note especially the end of the left big toe.

5

Differential Diagnosis

Causes Local to the Musculoskeletal System

In the foot there are six anatomical structures, namely: (1) bone and its periosteum; (2) hyaline cartilage; (3) the synovial capsules; (4) ligaments and retinacula; (5) muscles and their tendons and tendon sheaths; and (6) bursae. These may be the seat of one of five pathological changes which are: (1) changes due to trauma; (2) inflammatory conditions; (3) neoplastic conditions; (4) changes due to metabolic disease; and (5) congenital anomalies. In the foot, in addition to the musculoskeletal structures, the skin and fascia are also unusually frequent sources of pain because of pathological changes in them.

Not all of these structures are subject to all of these pathological changes; in fact, there are quite limited possibilities in differential diagnosis of the cause of pain in the foot arising from the structures of the musculoskeletal system.

Periosteum and Bone. TRAUMA. Any superficial bone can have its periosteum bruised by direct trauma. This is more likely to happen in the foot when the patient is going about barefooted. The sesamoids, having no periosteum, are spared from this.

Any bone can be fractured by trauma and sometimes simply by stress. In the foot two bones in particular may be the site of

82

stress fractures: the neck of a metatarsal bone (Fig. 5-1) and the calcaneus. Figure 5–2 shows a gross fracture of the calcaneus. It is included to demonstrate the change in the angle subtended by the long axis of the talus and that of the calcaneus which is normally about 35 degrees. Any angle less than this is suggestive of a fracture, and the diminution of the angle may be the only clue to the presence of an otherwise unidentifiable stress fracture of this bone. Compare the normal angle in Figure 5-6 for instance. These two stress fractures and a fracture through the waist of the talus are among those which classically may not

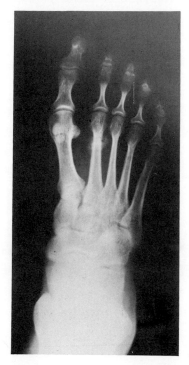

FIGURE 5-1. Stress fracture of the neck of the second metatarsal bone of the right foot. It was caused 3 weeks previously when the foot was struck against a stair. No evidence of fracture was seen in the original x-rays. Note the bipartite medial sesamoid on the right.

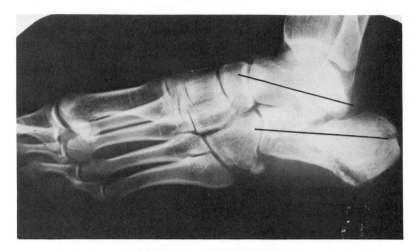

FIGURE 5-2. Gross fracture of the calcaneus, illustrating the loss of
the normal 35-degree angle subtended by lines drawn through the
long axis of the talus and calcaneus. The diminution of this angle
may be the only clue initially to the presence of a stress fracture.
Compare with the normal angle in Figure 5-6A.

be revealed radiographically until several days after the injury.
It is useful to remember that aspirated blood from a hematoma
in the area of trauma is diagnostic of a fracture if it contains fat
that is visible to the naked eye.

Osteochondritis juvenilis and aseptic necrosis following trauma
occur in the bones of the foot. Osteochondritis occurs classically
in the tarsal navicula which is called Köhler's disease (Fig. 5-3),
and in the head of the second metatarsal bone, which is called
Freiberg's disease (Fig. 5-4). Figure 5-5 illustrates osteochondritis dissecans of the medial superior aspect of the talus; ankle
pain was present for a considerable time before the diagnosis was
made. I have also seen this condition in a sesamoid bone produce
great pain and disability; the pathologist's report left some doubt
whether the pathological condition was osteochondritis or chondromalacia. Figures 5-6A through 5-6D illustrate this patient's

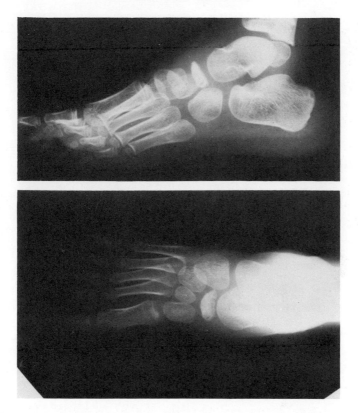

FIGURE 5-3. Typical x-ray appearance of osteochondritis of the tarsal navicula (Köhler's disease) in a child.

feet. Figure 5-7 illustrates a patient with osteochondritis of the lateral sesamoid. Sudeck's atrophy (Fig. 5-8) may ocur in the bones of the feet following trauma or immobilization (or both).

INFLAMMATION. Any bone of the foot may become the seat of hematogenous osteomyelitis of pyogenic (Fig. 5-9) or granulomatous etiology (Fig. 5–10). The bones may become infected by direct means in the presence of a compound fracture or following a puncture wound. The bones may be the seat of infarcts.

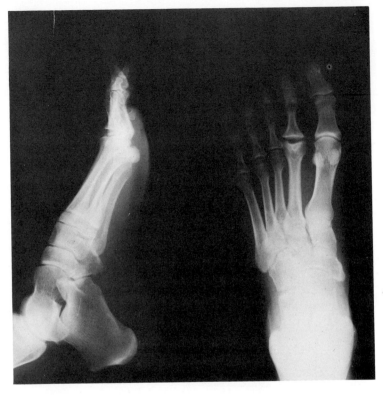

FIGURE 5-4.   Osteochondritis of the head of the second metatarsal
bone (Freiberg's disease).

NEOPLASMS.   The bones of the feet may be the seat of primary benign or malignant tumors. Figure 5-11 illustrates Kaposi's
sarcoma. Figures 5-12 and 5-13 illustrate benign osteochondro-
mas. I have never seen the bones of the feet invaded by metastases,
but there is no reason why this should not occur.

METABOLIC DISEASE.   Metabolic disease of bone is a pain-
producing condition, and the bones of the feet may be affected
and cause symptoms.

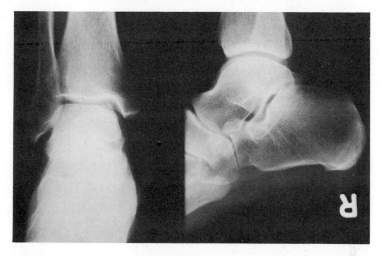

FIGURE 5-5.   Osteochondritis dissecans of the medial superior aspect of the talus. Ankle pain was present for a considerable time before the diagnosis was made.

CONGENITAL ANOMALIES.   Congenital anomalies of bones (Fig. 5-14), especially in relation to the navicula, talus, and calcaneus, cause painful "spastic" flatfeet. The congenital condition of prehallux may be a cause of pain. Morton's atavistic foot is a basis of pain from faulty weight bearing because of the congenital anomaly. Figure 5-15A illustrates the congenital anomaly of an extra ossification center at the base of the fifth metatarsal bone. Figure 5-15B illustrates separation of the extra ossification center following trauma.

Hyaline Cartilage. TRAUMA.   Hyaline cartilage, having no nerve supply, cannot itself be a seat of pain. However, if it is worn away or destroyed and bone is left rubbing on bone, then pain will ensue. Such a condition results from repetitive trauma. Chondral fractures may occur.

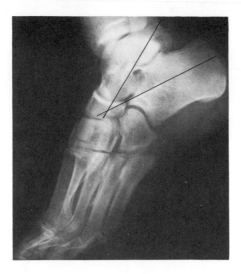

FIGURE 5-6A. An x-ray showing migration of the medial sesamoid bone under the head of the metatarsophalangeal joint of the big toe. (See also Figures 5-6B, 5-6C, and 5-6D.) The pathological report favored a diagnosis of chondromalacia. Note the normal 35-degree angle subtended by the long axis of the talus with the long axis of the calcaneus; compare with Figure 5-2, in which the calcaneus is fractured.

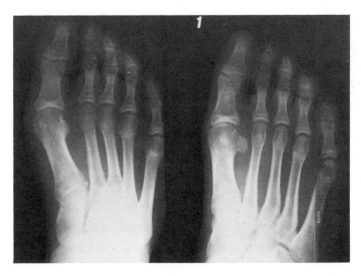

FIGURE 5-6B. Earlier x-rays of the same foot before migration of the medial sesamoid bone occurred. At this time the foot was very painful and swollen.

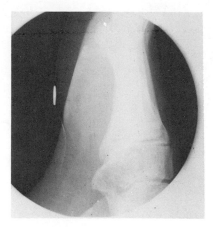

FIGURE 5-6C.   X-ray of the same foot showing early migration of the medial sesamoid bone and the associated soft tissue swelling.

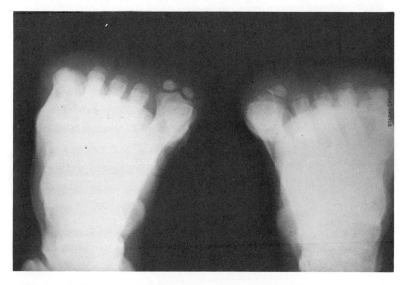

FIGURE 5-6D.   Tangential x-ray view of the patient's two feet clearly showing the pathological state of the medial sesamoid on the right.

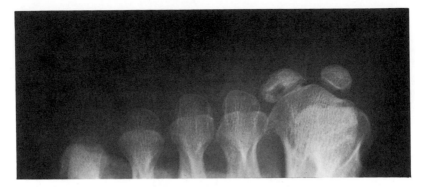

FIGURE 5-7.   Osteochondritis of the lateral sesamoid bone in another patient.

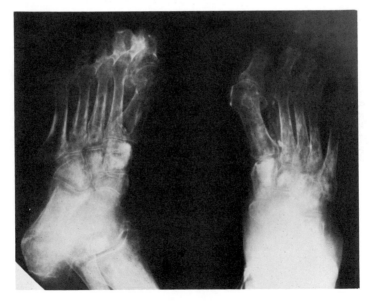

FIGURE 5-8.   Gross bone atrophy of the Sudeck type.

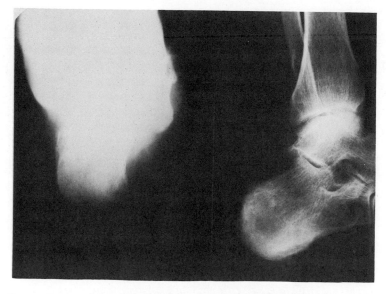

FIGURE 5-9. Osteomyelitis of the calcaneus. Symptoms of pain and swelling preceded the x-ray changes by many weeks.

INFLAMMATION. Hyaline cartilage is rapidly destroyed by blood or pus, and therefore pain may result from this, together with capsular inflammation. Osteochondritis dissecans (Fig. 5-5) may be an underlying cause of pain; if a loose piece of cartilage separates into the joint, pain and locking ensue.

Synovial Capsule. TRAUMA. Probably most pain from a joint arises from involvement of the synovial capsule. When traumatized, synovitis follows within 24 hours. If the trauma is more severe, hemarthrosis may result, the latter being far more painful than the former though the swelling is likely to be less.

GANGLION. Ganglia are quite common since the advent of surfing. The ganglia of a surfer's foot have to be seen to be be-

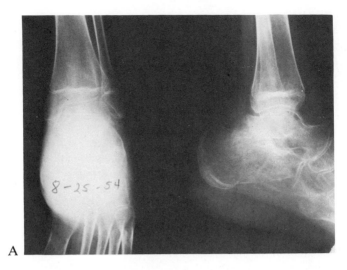

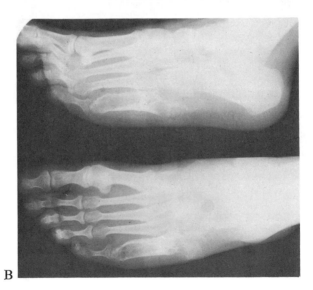

FIGURE 5-10.   Tuberculosis of the subtalar joint (A) and of the fifth metatarsal bone (B). Again symptoms preceded the diagnosis by many weeks. The gross osteoporosis involving all the bones suggests the etiology. With osteomyelitis (Fig. 5-9) osteoporosis is often not such a marked feature.

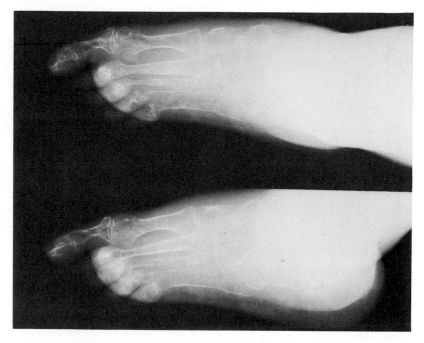

FIGURE 5-11. Kaposi's sarcoma. The patient had been under treatment for ulcers of both feet for some time before the diagnosis was made.

lieved (Fig. 5-16). Malignant changes have been reported in them, and they should not be regarded lightly. If one remembers that the capsule of a normal joint can never be palpated, a palpable capsule always suggests some serious pathological condition.

INFLAMMATION. Though in the true sense of the word blood in a joint sets up an inflammatory reaction of the synovium, in this context pyarthrosis is the topic of discussion. In the foot the condition may follow a puncture wound or be iatrogenic.

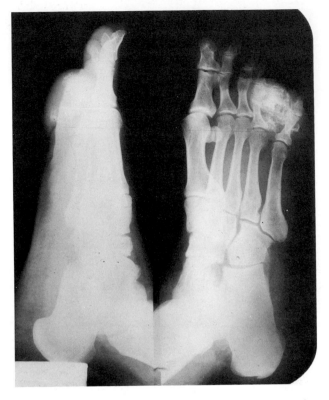

FIGURE 5-12.   A large osteochondroma originally presenting as a
painful soft tissue swelling under the fourth and fifth toes.

NEOPLASM.   The synovial capsule is a common seat of neoplastic changes. The synovioma is highly malignant. Mixed malignant tumors occur. Of the benign tumors, osteochrondroma-
tosis is probably most common; giant cell tumors and xanthomas
may be found, but they more commonly arise in the tendon
sheaths. Figure 5-17 is an x-ray of an advanced synovioma. The
original symptoms of swelling and pain were noted in June, 1949.
The diagnosis was not made until August, 1950, when ampu-
tation was performed. Lung metastases developed in 1954, and

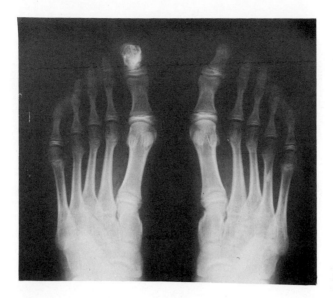

FIGURE 5-13. Osteochondroma of the distal phalanx of the left big toe (anteroposterior view).

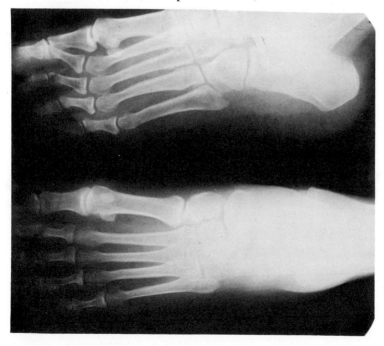

FIGURE 5-14. Congenital talocalcaneal bar.

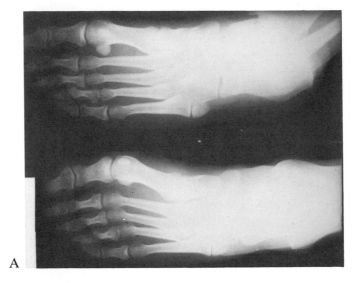

A

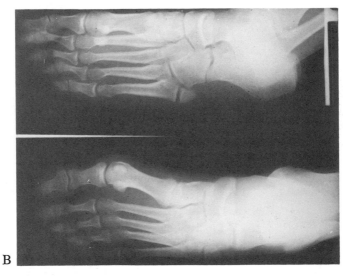

B

FIGURE 5-15.   A. Congenital extra ossification center at the base of the fifth metatarsal bone called the os vesalianum pedis. B. Separation of the os vesalianum following trauma, causing severe pain and prolonged disability. This might have been avoided had the patient been treated initially by using Goldthwaite strapping (Fig. 6-2B).

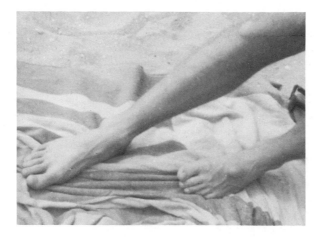

FIGURE 5-16. Surfer's feet showing typical ganglia. Malignant changes have been reported in them, and they should not be regarded lightly. (Note ganglion just below right knee.) (Courtesy of Tim Dorsey.)

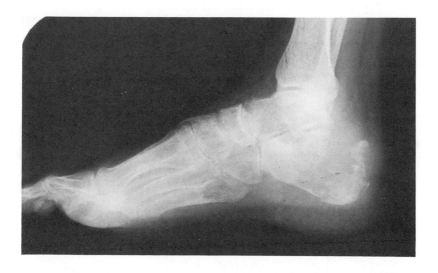

FIGURE 5-17. Synovioma which remained undiagnosed for nearly 14 months after symptoms of pain and swelling started.

the patient died in 1955. Somewhere between neoplasm and in-flammation comes the condition of pigmented villonodular syno-vitis, which is locally invasive but not metastatic.

Ligaments. TRAUMA.   Ligaments are a common seat of pain from joints. It must be remembered that ligaments are never ten-der on palpation unless the ligament itself is injured or there is something wrong with the joint which the ligament supports. Ligaments may be stretched (strained) by trauma, ligamentous fibers may be torn, or the ligament may be ruptured. A ruptured ligament is probably a more serious injury than a fracture. The diagnosis is made by demonstrating abnormal, excessive move-ment and proved by using stress x-rays. Figure 5-18 shows trac-ings from x-rays of the same ankle. A, without stress, reveals no injury. B, with stress, demonstrates rupture of the deltoid liga-ment by virtue of the tilted talus.

Muscles (Tendons and Tendon Sheaths). TRAUMA.   Muscles may be contused or sprained or have their fibers torn and their

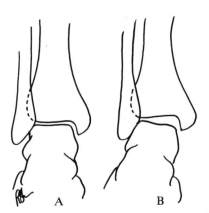

FIGURE 5-18.   Tilting of the talus in the mortise in x-ray tracings. This is diagnostic of rupture of a collateral ligament and would be missed were not adequate stress used to demonstrate the tilt.

tendons ruptured. If a tendon sheath is injured, traumatic tenosynovitis may result.

INFLAMMATION. The inflammatory conditions of muscle which cause pain are pathologically somewhat nebulous but clinically very real. These are fibro(myo)sitis and tendinitis. By the term *fibrositis* is meant a condition in which there is diffuse infiltration of muscle by a nonspecific inflammatory process characterized by painful localized nodules with areas of round cell infiltration. The cause is thought to be secondary either to a distant focus of infection or to impaired removal of catabolites because of lack of physiological muscle pumping from, for instance, unrelieved muscle spasm which itself may result from another cause of muscle pain or from reflex splinting to prevent pain from another structure. Tendinitis indicates a degenerative inflammatory condition of a muscle tendon, usually from mechanical attrition and overfunction. Tenosynovitis may be a reaction to nonspecific low-grade inflammation, possibly following trauma, or may herald more serious disease such as a collagen vascular disease or tuberculosis and cannot, therefore, be regarded lightly. The myopathies, atrophies, and dystrophies in themselves are not painful, but in the foot pain may result because joint structures become overused in compensating for the loss of muscle support.

NEOPLASM. Neoplasms of muscle are uncommon and often malignant, and may be of mixed type. Benign neoplasms of tendon sheaths, such as giant cell tumor and xanthoma, may be found. They can be the seat of malignant neoplasms. Figure 5-19 illustrates a giant cell tumor of a tendon sheath.

CONGENITAL ANOMALY. Muscles are sometimes absent from birth; this may result in loss of function and in the development

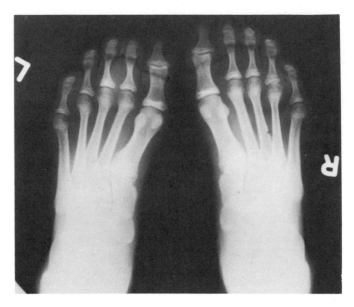

FIGURE 5-19.   Giant cell tumor of tendon sheath indicated by soft
tissue swelling in relation to the second and third toes of the left
foot.

of pain. They may be inadequate following the correction of other
congenital anomalies; pain may arise from the resulting strain
and loss of normal physiological function.

Bursae

TRAUMA.   A nonspecific traumatic bursitis is not uncommon,
and in the foot may be acute or chronic. The presence of bursitis,
however, may herald systemic disease such as collagen vascular
disease and gout.

INFLAMMATION AND NEOPLASMS.   Bursae may be involved
in acute inflammatory processes for reasons other than trauma.

In that bursae are lined by synovium, they can be the source of neoplasms.

Joint Dysfunction. In addition to these well-accepted and well-documented pathological conditions which occur in the musculoskeletal system and produce pain, "joint dysfunction," a mechanical cause of pain, is probably the single commonest cause of pain arising from joints which are subject to unguarded movement, immobilization, or disuse or following the resolution of any other pathological condition. Frequently, the joints in the foot are mechanically impaired by loss of their normal functional movement, resulting in loss of joint play and pain from joint dysfunction.

Causes Not Local to the Musculoskeletal System

It has been pointed out in the foregoing section that even causes of pain which appear to be local to the musculoskeletal system may in fact be the heralding manifestation of systemic disease. Examples of this were noted in tenosynovitis, which may be a manifestation of collagen vascular disease or tuberculosis, and in bursitis, which may be a manifestation of collagen vascular disease or gout.

Systemic Disease. There are a multitude of other causes of musculoskeletal pain in which the prime cause is not local to the musculoskeletal structures themselves but is due to systemic diseases. The foot is not spared from such painful manifestations of these diseases.

Pain in the foot which appears to be involving a joint or joints may indicate the presence of rheumatic fever or any of the collagen vascular diseases — that is, rheumatoid arthritis, Reiter's syndrome, psoriatic arthritis, scleroderma, dermatomyositis, lupus erythematosus, and polymyositis.

Symptoms of bone and joint pain may be associated with pulmonary disease, congenital cardiac conditions, or kidney disease; joint pain may be associated with Henoch's purpura and other hemorrhagic dyscrasias, most especially hemophilia. Arthralgia may be associated with acromegaly and ulcerative colitis.

The joints of the feet are no more free from involvement by tuberculosis, gout, brucellosis, sarcoidosis, allergic serositis, and nonspecific intermittent hydrarthrosis than any other joint.

With the recent wars and the general increase in travel, one may expect an unusual influx of patients with joint involvement from amebiasis, fungal infections, hydatid disease, yaws, leprosy, and other tropical diseases. Echinococciasis and trichinosis may enjoy a recrudescence.

Syphilis and gonorrhea also affect the joints. Gonococcal arthritis is exquisitely painful, and syphilitic involvement of the synovium (Clutton's joint) or the bone-cartilage complex (Charcot's joint) is by no means painless in the early stages.

Skin and Fascial Structures. In addition to local musculoskeletal causes of pain and those arising from systemic diseases, in the foot we have in addition causes of pain resulting from its rather specialized integument — the skin and fascial structures.

CALLOSITIES AND CORNS. Corns are a localized form of callosity, the designation being interchangeable. Corns are often divided into two types — the dry and the wet. This is probably an artificial differentiation, and a wet corn, being between the toes, is probably the same as a dry one but softened by moisture from poor foot care.

A callous is simply a reactive hyperplasia of the skin produced by irritation from without or within or a combination of both. They are usually normal and act as a perfect self-made protective slipper. There is no reason for interfering with them unless the overgrowth is excessive and a very obvious cause of difficulty when the foot is shod. They are particularly found under the metatarsal heads in feet in which there is unevenness of weight bearing and are nature's way of protecting the sensitive head of the bone. They develop from rubbing the skin on roughened ridges of, or perhaps a protruding nail in, the insole of shoes.

PLANTAR WARTS (VERRUCAE PLANTARIS). Although plantar warts microscopically resemble thickened corns, it is thought that they have a viral etiology. They are papillomatous structures with excessive thickening of the epidermis and cornification of the surface layers of the skin. It is the thickened epithelium pressing on sensory nerve endings which causes the pain. These warts have a fibrous core, with marked connective tissue overgrowth surrounding it. When the superficial layers of epithelium are removed, the wart reveals its demarked nature which differentiates it from a corn.

ATHLETE'S FOOT (EPIDERMOPHYTOSIS). This condition, a fungal infection of the skin, is very common. Starting usually between the toes, it may spread widely throughout the sole of the foot and be a cause of severe foot pain.

CHILBLAINS, TRENCH FOOT, IMMERSION FOOT. Although these three entities primarily are due to vascular involvement, their manifestations are largely superficial and in the skin.

Chilblains (lupus pernio) occur from exposure to cold, with or without a wet environment, which results in dermatitis and sometimes ulceration of the skin. There is associated perivascular infiltration and intimal proliferation. Subcutaneous tissues and the skin show a chronic inflammatory reaction with giant cells, and there may be fat necrosis.

Trench foot results from exposure to a wet, cold environment also, but exposure is more prolonged and the cold often less intense. Immobility or the wearing of constrictive foot gear may play a part. Trench foot can be very painful. Characteristically the foot is swollen, there are skin blebs, and the papillary vessels are dilated. Hyperhidrosis may be a feature, and sludging of the blood may occur, with resulting thrombosis and maybe gangrene.

Immersion foot is similar to trench foot, but the wet environment seems to be more important than the cold; it may occur with relatively warm immersion. Clinically, there are two stages — vasoconstriction and hyperemia. In the latter stage there is erythema, edema, vesiculation, and sometimes gangrene. Sensory loss is common because of nerve involvement. Motor paralysis may be a feature.

FROSTBITE.   Frostbite is not very different from the foregoing conditions, but etiologically the exposure to cold does not have to be associated with exposure to wetness. The cold in this condition has to be below freezing, and the amount of damage varies with the intensity of the cold and the duration of exposure. If the circulation is impaired at the time of exposure, the damage will be proportionately greater. There is early vasoconstriction followed by dilatation. The vessel walls become thickened and the vessel lumen is partially or completely occluded. Edema of the cutis occurs. Vascular thrombosis with tissue necrosis follows, and secondary infection may become a complication. Nerve involvement may occur.

PLANTAR FASCIITIS. This is a painful condition of the plantar fascia, probably due to its overstretching on ambulation and to constant repetitive trauma. It has a counterpart in Ober's syndrome, a painful fibrotic reaction in the iliotibial bands. It is a very real cause of foot pain.

DUPUYTREN'S CONTRACTURE. This is the same condition as that found in the palmar fascia of the hand and results in a progressive constriction of the plantar fascia with contracture and pain. It may be a more acute manifestation of plantar fasciitis. It does not respond to conservative treatment.

SOFTENING OF THE SOLES OF THE FEET. Following immobilization in plaster or illness requiring prolonged bed rest, the soles of the feet atrophy as do the subcutaneous fat pads. Little attention is paid to this, and on resuming ambulation the unfortunate patient has no protection, particularly under the heads of the metatarsal bones which become readily traumatized and a source of considerable pain iatrogenically induced and unnecessary. Even lay people in the infantry and the sports field know better than this and take steps to "toughen up" the feet of the new recruit. Just plain blisters may be a cause of severe foot pain, and if they become secondarily infected, the problem is compounded.

CONTRACTURE OF ACHILLES TENDON AND PLANTAR FASCIA. Under the same circumstances as those leading to softening of the soles of the feet and atrophy of the fat pads, especially if there is any degree of plantar flexion of the foot in plaster or if the bed clothes are tightly tucked in over the invalid's feet, the Achilles tendons and the plantar fascia, and, for that matter, all the fascial sheaths, contract to a marked degree in a very short time. This results in an insufficiency of the Achilles tendons which, by itself, produces an unnatural drop of the forefoot; this is compounded by the loss of resiliency, particularly of the plantar fascia. Together or separately these conditions alter the mechanics of the feet in weight bearing and become a potent cause of foot pain. This is further aggravated when the patient is allowed to resume walking in heelless, ill-fitting bedroom slippers; if supplied by a hospital, these are often no more than paper foot coverings which are worse still.

Vascular and Neurogenic Causes of Foot Pain. Symptoms of pain due to vascular and neurogenic causes are for some reason more prevalent in the feet than in any other part of either extremity.

ARTERIAL DISEASE. Intermittent claudication pain or muscle cramps, which may be excruciatingly painful, characterize insufficiency or disease of the vascular system. The feet are a common seat of these symptoms of pain. It is not a criterion of arterial disease that the pulses must be absent. Angiospasm itself is painful, and the pain may simply be due to the spasm of transient ischemia. Ischemic neuritis is probably a vasoneuropathy. It is associated with numbness, aching, burning, paresthesia, and frank pain. It is not uncommon with diabetes, syphilis, thromboangiitis obliterans, and arteriosclerotic disease. Though the cause of the neuritic element differs in each disease, the effect is the same to all intents and purposes.

In diabetes, in addition to ischemia of the nerve trunks primarily, there is a degeneration of the nerves which is greater in proportion to the amount of arterial disease present and, to this extent, may be unrelated to the vascular deficiency. In thromboangiitis obliterans the neuritis, due to an inflammatory reaction involving the nerve trunks which aggravates the ischemic element, seems to be caused purely by ischemia.

Syphilis primarily attacks the posterior nerve roots, though there is an associated ischemia and the pains resulting are characterized as "lightning pains."

Erythromelalgia is a functional vascular disease associated with burning pain and redness of the feet, often with swelling. The cause is uncertain but seems to result from loss of vasomotor control or from dysfunction of the sympathetic nervous system. There certainly appears to be a change of sensitivity in the skin to heat. It may be primary, or it may be a complication of other vascular diseases and diseases such as gout, hemiplegia, polycythemia, and multiple sclerosis. Raynaud's disease may affect the feet and be the cause of foot pain. It involves particularly the digital arteries and arterioles.

VENOUS CAUSES. Foot pain may be a symptom of venous disease either from venous insufficiency or in the presence of venous thrombosis, especially deep-vein thrombosis. The differentiation of venous disease pain from arterial disease pain is sometimes difficult; however, pain from venous causes tends to improve with elevation of the part, whereas that from arterial disease tends to be aggravated by elevation. Venous disease pain does not have the intermittent characteristic of arterial claudication.

PSEUDOINTERMITTENT CLAUDICATION. This arises from an insufficiency of the Achilles tendons in patients who wear shoes with insufficiently high heels. The pain may be in the feet or the legs (or both) and is probably due to a mechanical ischemia from stretching of the gastrocnemius-soleus group of muscles which occludes to varying degrees the vascular tree on walking and running. Its differentiation from organic intermittent claudication is important as it is so easily treated by proper adaptation of the heel height of footwear.

NEUROGENIC CAUSES.   Morton's neuroma is a classic cause of foot pain. The neuroma is usually found at the decussation of the digital nerve between the heads of the third and fourth metatarsal bones. However, a neuroma may also be found similarly situated between the second and third digits in patients with a congenital syndactyly between these toes. It is of passing interest that the Morton who described the neuroma is not the person referred to in the term *Morton's foot*.

Paresthesia in the foot or pain in the foot may herald the onset of neurological disease. Thus a patient presenting painful feet merits a complete neurological examination. Dysfunction of the autonomic nervous system may also be a cause of foot pain. Sudeck's bone atrophy in the foot does not respond as well to sympathetic block as it does to stellate ganglion block in the hand. A disk prolapse in the back can manifest itself solely as foot pain.

Other Causes of Foot Pain.   LYMPHATIC DISEASE.   Foot pain may arise from disease of the lymphatic system but is acute only in the presence of acute lymphangitis which has obvious clinical features. Aching pain is associated with chronic lymphatic obstruction which is characterized by nonpitting edema.

MUSCLE CRAMPS.   Muscle cramps may produce severe foot pain and may or may not be due to vascular disease. Pain from them may last for minutes or maybe days, though the cramp itself may be transient. When the cramps are secondary to vascular disease, other manifestations of these diseases are present. They may also be associated with venous or lymphatic diseases as well as arterial diseases. Cramps occurring without vascular disease may result from mechanical ischemia from fatigue of the muscles of the feet whose physiological state is poorly maintained.

However, cramps may be associated with diseases manifesting various metabolic aberrations, and their differential diagnosis is important. They may occur in patients on salt-free diets in hot weather or from the abuse of diuretic medications with excessive loss of electrolytes or from deficient chloride intake; they are analogous to miner's cramps of the past.

CEREBRAL PALSY. Foot deformities may arise in cerebral palsy patients, but normally corrective treatment is undertaken in youth. Pes cavus from a contracted Achilles tendon and deformity from peroneal spasm may result in pain in later life. Treatment has to vary with the cause of pain, and not necessarily the obvious deformity.

CHARCOT-MARIE-TOOTH DISEASE. In a similar way pain may result from the pes cavus deformity which occurs with peroneal muscular atrophy. In this condition the development of pain may be avoided by the wearing of special shoes from the time that the deformity becomes apparent. Exercise programs in this condition are contraindicated because the primary muscle pathology is irreversible and progressive.

ROCKER BOTTOM FOOT. The rocker bottom foot resulting from mismanagement of the clubfoot is an insoluble problem using conservative measures.

CALCANEAL OSTEOCHONDRITIS. This is a problem which causes pain in the heel of the foot in adolescents and hardly falls into the scope of this work as it is usually self-limiting. Unlike the other osteochondritic conditions, it does not cause symptoms in late life. However, improperly resolved, it might be an underlying cause of foot pain from an unduly short Achilles tendon; treatment would follow the principles outlined for treatment of Achilles tendon insufficiency.

6

Common Causes of Foot Pain and Their Treatment

Bone and Joint Pain

"Metatarsalgia."   *Metatarsalgia* is a generic term for pain in and around the heads of the metatarsal bones with no underlying pathological changes. Treatment for metatarsalgia, then, must at best be empirical, and so often must be fruitless. First it is necessary to define the pathological conditions that give rise to this pain, and then discuss the rational and specific treatment for each condition.

JOINT DYSFUNCTION.   There are no true synovial joints between the heads of the metatarsal bones, so there cannot be joint dysfunction between them in the pure sense of the term. However, there are small bursae between them which, when traumatized and swollen, are painful. With their chronic irritation from being constantly crushed together by shoes that are too tight across the metatarsal heads, adherence between bone, bursa, and bone becomes established. Also, the ligaments of the metatarsophalangeal joints in their lateral aspects become tender from trauma. Finally, the intermetatarsal ligaments become fibrotic, and any stretching of them becomes painful. The pain (metatar-

111

salgia) resulting from these multiple causes and complicated by joint dysfunction is very severe. Any schoolboy knows how to imitate the pain by crushing the heads of the metacarpal bones together with a hard, twisting type of handshake, and does it for fun.

Treatment.   Mobilization of both the metatarsal heads (see pages 59–62) and the metatarsophalangeal joints (see pages 55–59) and ensuring that the patient wears wide enough shoes (measuring for this as described on pages 217, 232) are often sufficient to relieve metatarsalgia from these causes completely. In very chronic and severe cases it is also necessary to fit a metatarsal-head support, as described on pages 213–215, and to treat the muscles of the foot (both intrinsic and extrinsic) by faradic foot baths (page 172), exercise (pages 174–175), and massage (page 173).

SHORT ACHILLES TENDON.   Almost as severe metatarsal-head pain is experienced by patients who have Achilles tendon insufficiency; this condition is often associated with plantar fasci-itis because of the chronic exaggerated drop of the forefoot. In this condition, to put the ball of the foot on the ground at the same time as the heel, the front part of the foot goes into eversion; the forefoot also is usually flail. In this everted position the heads of the metatarsal bones spread unduly, stretching the inter-metatarsal ligaments and thus causing more pain in addition to that resulting from weight bearing on the wrong aspects of the metatarsal heads.

Treatment.   In its less severe forms, compensation for the insufficiency of the Achilles tendon by building up the heel of the shoe as described on page 200, together with a snug, supporting fit of the shoe width just behind the metatarsal heads, is usually sufficient. In more severe cases, platform supports must be fashioned to support the inner aspect of the foot and to redistribute the weight bearing on the metatarsal heads. In such severe cases, mobilization of all the joints of the foot may be necessary, and the musculature almost certainly requires treatment as well.

(D. J.) MORTON'S ATAVISTIC FOOT. In this condition, whatever the primary problem, the second metatarsal bone is longer than that of the big toe (measured from the sesamoid bones) and its shaft is thicker than the shafts of the metatarsal bones of the third, fourth, and fifth toes. (Usually there is little difference in the width of the four lateral metatarsal shafts.) This broadening and overdevelopment of the metatarsal shaft is surely caused by the second metatarsal bone taking an undue amount of the stresses of weight bearing. To use the term *atavism* properly, one must accept that the big toe is short and deflected into varus. A big toe in congenital varus is often found clinically to be in valgus deformity to some degree. This is because a shoe that is too short has a toe cap that swerves out proximally to the first metatarsophalangeal joint and pushes the big toe into valgus. This may give rise to permanent deformity.

A callus is frequently present under the head of the second metatarsal bone — nature's attempt to save it from the trauma and unnatural stress that it was never designed to bear. The callus itself is painful, and indeed may be a painful corn.

Treatment. This condition can be effectively relieved only by fashioning a well-fitting metatarsal-head support and by ensuring adequate width of the forepart of the shoe to accommodate the varus of the big toe. Invariably there is some degree of joint dysfunction in the related joints, which must be relieved by mobilization.

(T. G.) MORTON'S NEUROMA. The "metatarsalgia" from a digital neuroma, usually between the fourth and fifth toes at the level of the metatarsal heads deep in the plantar aspect of the foot, is among the most acutely painful conditions of the foot. The pain may radiate anywhere in the foot. The neuroma is usually palpable, and when squeezed, the acute knife-like pain is reproduced.

Treatment. To remove the neuroma is simple, quick, and sure. Small digital areas of numbness may remain. However, following surgery, joint mobilization and muscle treatment should be undertaken. The pain from the neuroma has produced widespread muscle spasm that probably has caused secondary fibrositis in the intrinsic muscles, and almost certainly has produced joint dysfunction by splinting of the joints. Both of these conditions help to maintain residual symptoms.

PLANTAR WART. A similar acute, shooting, lancinating neuroma-like pain may be caused by a plantar wart. There should be no difficulty in diagnosis since the wart can be easily seen on the sole of the foot.

Treatment. Treatment of a plantar wart may be very frustrating. Kent and Bender, and Leonard et al. have reported on the successful use of ultrasound, but I have not been particularly impressed with its efficiency. It has the merit of being easy to apply, however, and is, I believe, innocuous if it fails.

The vesicant Cantharone has given favorable results.

Chemical cauterization by salicylic acid up to 60% strength and electrocauterization are effective. When salicylic acid is used, the keratotic skin associated with the plantar wart should be first pared down. Isolated plantar warts can then be excised.

However, carelessness in proper sterile surgical technique, particularly in cleansing of the skin, has not infrequently been the cause of the loss of a limb, especially in a diabetic patient. In recalcitrant cases x-ray therapy or the application of radium by an experienced radiotherapist is often successful.

CALLOSITIES AND CORNS.   Corns, which are really local callosities, are usually found under the weight-bearing heads of the metatarsal bones or over the phalangeal knuckles. Metatarsalgia from corns may be very severe. On examination the immediate cause is very apparent, but the cause of the cause is almost always overlooked; also, the treatment by paring, corn plasters, chemical cautery, excision (see under plantar warts for inherent dangers) can only be symptomatic.

Treatment.   Shoes should be inspected for protruding nails and ridges. If it is noted that shoe stitching passes over the location of the callus or corn and the shoe is particularly rigid in such areas, this must be changed. The so-called soft corn is usually between the toes. The involved toes rub together because of either shoe pressure from an unsuitable toe cap or overlapping or otherwise distorted toes. Correction of these things will relieve pain arising from a callus, which should then disappear. However, the callus or corn that produces metatarsalgia is usually caused by faulty weight bearing over one or other of the lateral four metatarsal heads. This can be cured only by using a properly fashioned metatarsal-head support. Mobilization of the relating joints relieves residual pain.

SIMPLE HALLUX VALGUS.   Hallux valgus may cause no symptoms. When it is painful, a very common cause of the pain is traumatic joint dysfunction in the first metatarsophalangeal joint. If the "trauma" is more severe, chronic traumatic arthritis and synovitis of that joint occur. A dorsal exostosis is often associated with this. The pain may largely be due to improper weight bearing on the metatarsal heads because of the hallux deformity. The pain may also be arising from an associated bunion.

Treatment.   Treatment of the joint dysfunction in the first metatarsophalangeal joint by manipulation often affords the patient dramatic relief of pain. This relief can be maintained if the toe of the shoe is broad enough not to press inward on the digit and the metatarsal head. Early osteoarthritic changes are of no significance and do not contraindicate mobilization therapy or lessen its usefulness.

If, however, there is dorsal subchondral bony hypertrophic lipping, mobilization will probably fail. Then an anterior metatarsal-head support is necessary to relieve the first metatarsal head of weight bearing and the first metatarsophalangeal joint of some dorsiflexion in walking. If the hallux valgus is part of an atavistic foot, treatment follows the plan already described on page 113.

The development of a painful bunion can be prevented by proper design of the front of the shoes, with care to ensure that there is no stitching or brogue work anywhere near the metatarsophalangeal joint and that no toe cap is incorporated in the shoe. A Blucher shoe made on a cantilever or straight last is the shoe of choice.

HALLUX RIGIDUS.   If literally the hallux were rigid at the metatarsophalangeal joint, as the term implies, there could be no metatarsalgia associated with it; clinically, the joint would be fused, which is not the case. Hallux rigidus is just a more severe form of hallux valgus. Usually marked changes of traumatic arthritis as well as associated capsular and ligamentous changes are present in the metatarsophalangeal joint. A bunion (acute or chronic bursitis) over the medial aspect of the deformed joint is almost always an added problem.

Treatment.   Though this is a condition which perhaps is best treated by surgery, even this will fail unless full foot rehabilitation follows and unless proper shoes are prescribed after surgery. Very adequate relief, however, can be obtained from the pain of this condition by physical therapy and foot care. Certainly when such a severe deformity is present on one joint, other joints in the foot are also involved. So the full regimen of foot care described in Chapter 8 must be carried out. Shoes can be designed to accommodate almost any deformity, but in this instance proper heel height may be especially important. To prevent painful movement of the deformed and diseased major joint, not only must a platform support (or at least a metatarsal-head support) be incorporated in the shoe, but a rocker bottom (sole) must also be built on the outside of the shoe. With this the shoe then takes up almost all the dorsiflexion which the joint otherwise has to accommodate in simple walking.

THE "BROKEN DOWN" FOOT.   This term describes the foot of the invalid or the patient who has had prolonged immobilization of the lower limb in plaster. The skin and underlying fat are atrophied and the fascia and ligaments have lost their elasticity and under some circumstances may be contracted or sometimes stretched. The muscles are atrophied from disuse, and their tendons may be contracted. The joints all show dysfunction from disuse and may even be partially "frozen." Finally the vascular supply is deficient and the lymph channels inefficient or even blocked. Attempted function produces diffuse metatarsalgia and every other "algia" known to the musculoskeletal system.

Treatment.   The full gamut of treatment as described in

Chapter 7 must be carried out with great patience and accuracy. When mobilization techniques are used as part of the program, a short leg plaster is applied after manipulation of the joints, as it is sometimes in the plaster correction of the feet in children, to "soften-up" the foot. But it is left on for only 2 days and then the full program is resumed.

THE "RHEUMATOID" FOOT.   In a patient with rheumatoid arthritis in whom the disease seems otherwise quiescent or in whom at least there are no other acute manifestations, there is often acute metatarsalgia which the rheumatologist often ascribes to the disease. In my experience this singular foot pain is so often caused by a mechanical dropping of the head of the fourth metatarsal bone, and less frequently the head of the third metatarsal bone, that it merits stress here as a cause of readily relievable symptoms. On examination there is an obvious mechanical downward displacement of the metatarsal head, which is acutely tender on palpation and on movement in relation to the adjacent metatarsal heads. There is no clinical evidence of acute inflammation such as local heat or joint swelling.

Treatment.   An anterior metatarsal-head support fashioned in the usual way (pages 213–215) is made, but a depression is hollowed out in the straight, beveled front edge on which the lateral four metatarsal heads rest to receive and cradle this one dropped metatarsal head.

If a rheumatoid patient also has atavism of the foot, the pain from this is usually not part of the disease but is due to the mechanical stresses of the abnormal foot. Pain symptoms from this are also readily treatable by the regimen described on page 113. The addition of Jacobson's relaxation therapy to any program of treatment prescribed for pain in rheumatoid arthritis is of enormous benefit to the patient as a whole and especially to the part being treated; thus it has a place in treating the painful rheumatoid foot.

Deformed Toes.   Feet with deformed toes would probably not be painful if these were not jammed into conventional footwear. Treatment of pain from this cause is to provide proper shoes.

OVERLAPPING TOES.   Overlapping toes can be corrected by taping of one sort or another designed to correct the overlap by tension or pressure (Fig. 6-1). No one technique is better than another, and anyone can design his own method as long as it achieves the desired mechanical effect. However, this treatment is a useless exercise unless proper shoes are prescribed. The details of proper shoe prescription are found in Chapter 11.

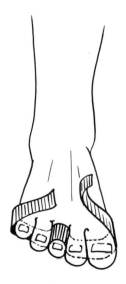

FIGURE 6-1.   The correction of an overlapping third toe by the use of tape.

CLAW TOES (HAMMER TOES).   This deformity does not fall into the province of this book, dealing as it does only with non-surgical forms of treatment. However, shoes can be designed to accommodate deformed toes of this kind, with resulting foot comfort.

CONGENITAL TOE ANOMALIES.   The same must be said for congenital toe deformities as for claw toes and hammer toes: The feet can be accommodated in special shoes. With syn-dactylism, especially when present between the second and third toes, a neuroma may be the cause of pain.

The commonest cause of foot pain associated with toe deformi-ties is the development of wet or dry corns resulting from irrita-tion of ill-fitting shoes and poor foot hygiene. Treatment for the relief of pain, therefore, must be directed at these conditions, too.

Congenital Foot Anomalies.   Congenital deformities of the feet and the lower extremity which may cause foot problems are the clubfoot or one of its individual components, either separately or in different combinations. These are a short Achilles tendon, metatarsus varus, and tarsus varus in the foot. Tibial torsion, femoral torsion, and antiversion of the hip in the upper part of the lower extremity may also lead to foot problems. These con-ditions are usually adequately cared for in infancy and childhood by the orthopedist and do not cause foot pain. If residual prob-lems remain untreated, however, they may be a cause of foot pain in later years; these patients usually can be relieved of their symp-toms only by the use of every part of the regimens of management that are discussed in Chapter 7.

ACCESSORY NAVICULA OR PREHALLUX.   In this condition the pain usually has a mechanical origin. The posterior tibial muscle makes its main insertion into the upper instead of the lower aspect of the navicula, thereby losing much of its supportive function and resulting in strain of the ligaments on the plantar aspect of the foot in the region of the talonavicular joint. In addition, traumatic tendinitis of the tibialis posterior may occur from misuse. Foot valgus may increase the strain.

Treatment. Though the Kidner operation is designed to correct the faults of this congenital anomaly, comfort may be obtained by wearing proper shoes with a well-designed platform support, by treatment of the traumatic tendinitis of the tibialis posterior muscle with ice massage, and by treating the various other strained components of the foot along the lines suggested for total foot care. Even after surgery, proper shoes and complete foot rehabilitation are a prerequisite to success of the operation.

PLANTAR LIGAMENT AND TARSAL JOINT LIGAMENT STRAIN. *Ligament and Fascia Pain.* Pain from ligaments and the plantar fascia almost always manifests itself in the plantar aspect of the foot. To differentiate between the pain from the plantar fascia and that from the long plantar and short plantar ligaments and from ligaments supporting the individual tarsal joints is especially difficult. The patient localizes the pain from each cause as being under the "longitudinal arch."

With plantar ligament strain, palpation will reveal localized tender areas at both the origin under the calcaneus and the insertion at the bases of the metatarsal bones. If the heads of the metatarsals are then pressed plantarward, the ligaments relax and the tender points in the long and short plantar ligaments become less tender. If, however, the reverse occurs, and there is little tenderness on palpation with the foot outstretched and increased tenderness on pressing the metatarsal heads plantarward, then the ligaments supporting the tarsal joints or tarsometatarsal joints are the source of the pain. Pain from plantar fasciitis differs from this picture only in that the fascia can be felt to be tight, pain is elicited on more superficial palpation, and the area that is painful to palpation is more diffuse and is noted in both positions of the foot equally.

Treatment. Treatment of ligament strain is rest from function, together with sedative physical therapy if the cause of the strain is acute. The physical therapy modalities may include whirlpool bath, in which free foot, toe, and ankle movement should be encouraged. Ultrasound, using small wattage, is conveniently given while the foot is in the water. Recovery should not take more than a few days, but on returning to active weight bearing, a temporary anterior metatarsal-head support made of felt should be worn for 4 to 6 weeks (see pages 213–215). If the ligament strain is so severe as to suggest that tearing of some fibers may have occurred, then the application of a plaster cast may have to precede the physical therapy program. In this case, a more comprehensive physical therapy program has to be used, including muscle reeducation as described on pages 172–175.

Treatment of plantar fasciitis is designed to try to soften and stretch the fascia. Rest from function is again a prerequisite to successful treatment. The use of a cast with the foot extended in its long axis may soften up the foot. Ultrasound has the property of softening scar tissue and is used underwater following whirlpool treatment. Massage and manual stretching after this helps. Usually one ends up prescribing a properly fashioned platform support (see pages 199–211) to avoid undue further stretching on the resumption of function. A Ripple Sole shoe is helpful to maintain comfort in cases of either ligament strain or fascia inflammation.

LIGAMENTS OF THE SUBTALAR JOINT. Sprains of the ligaments of the subtalar joint, which invariably complicate a severely twisted ankle, are almost certainly always associated with joint synovitis. After resolution of all the associated acute pathological manifestations, there is invariably residual subtalar joint dysfunction. Strain of the subtalar joint ligament is characterized by pain on palpation in the sinus tarsi. Mobilization of the joint is almost always required to relieve the residual pain symptoms.

DUPUYTREN'S CONTRACTURE.   Dupuytren's contracture in its early stages may easily be confused with simple plantar fasciitis. Careful palpation and the presence of tender, thickened nodules, especially under the instep, should suggest the correct diagnosis.

Treatment.   Ultrasound is said to be useful in treating this condition because of its property of softening fibrous tissue. In this condition, however, the proliferative fibroblastic hyperplasia, in conjunction with an active round cell infiltrative inflammatory process and its progressive course, mitigates against the success of any conservative treatment program.

Muscles and Tendons

FLEXOR HALLUCIS LONGUS TENDINITIS.   The tendon of the flexor hallucis longus is particularly prone to injury. The diagnosis is complicated by the fact that the most tender area of palpation is hard to distinguish from the tender ligament points described above. In this condition, however, there is no increased tenderness on palpation when the foot is moved from the rest position into the long axis extended position so long as the big toe is allowed to flex freely during the examining movement. If, in the extended position, the toe is now dorsiflexed, the pain is exacerbated and the whole tendon stands out and is found to be tender throughout its length. In these patients there is usually a depression in the insole of their shoes dug by the head of the first metatarsal bone.

Treatment.   The principle of treatment is to prevent constant stretching of this tendon. This can be achieved by raising the heel of the shoe, which must have a steel shank. Ice massage to the tendon and faradic foot baths, together with massage to the whole lower leg and relative rest from function during the acute phase, bring ready relief, though it may be necessary to add an anterior metatarsal-head support to new shoes to prevent the patient from having to dig a hole in the insole of the new shoe to accommodate the first metatarsal head.

OTHER EXTRINSIC MUSCLES.   Following injuries about the ankle or immobilization of the lower leg in plaster, any of the tendons of the extrinsic muscles may be strained or have their tendon sheaths injured or become adherent in the areas of the respective retinacula. Differential diagnosis can be made accurately only by palpation; when tenderness is localized, the suspected muscle has its function initiated and resisted and the pain will be aggravated when the right muscle is chosen. If tenosynovitis is the underlying pathological condition, crepitus is felt on movement of the muscle whose sheath is involved. The patient's pain symptoms may be appreciated in the foot in the areas through which the tendons course to their insertions. The insertion of the peroneus brevis is prone to avulsion, but then one is dealing with an avulsion fracture of the base of the fifth metatarsal bone which has to be treated as such.

Treatment.   Severe strain may have to be treated initially by immobilization, and even a plaster boot may have to be applied. Figure eight strapping, however, is often adequate if it is applied so that there is a pull of inversion or eversion under the instep (Fig. 6-2), depending on whether the strain involves

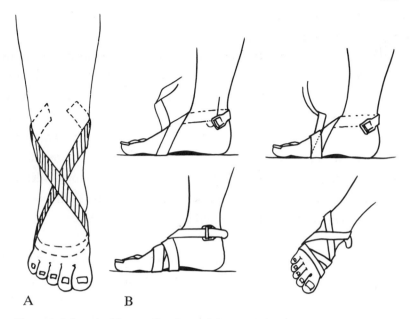

A   B

FIGURE 6-2.   A. The application of figure eight strapping for strain
of the muscles or ligaments on the medial or lateral side of the ankle.
B. Goldthwaite's strapping—a method especially suitable for treating
strain at the insertion of the peroneus brevis.

the muscles coursing around the medial or lateral malleolus.
Another very efficient way of achieving initial comfort is to soak
a gauze bandage in hot wax and then apply this by wrapping
around the foot and ankle. The heat, though transient, is com-
forting, and when the wax cools, it hardens to provide relieving
support. When the initial acute phase has settled down, treatment
by ice massage or vapor-coolant spray is as effective as any
treatment. Part of the skill involved in this therapy is to give
alternate stretching and relaxing movements to the involved muscle while the cooling counterirritant is being applied. Rest from
function until healing has occurred is a prerequisite to successful
therapy, as is attention to the whole lower leg rather than to the
involved tendon alone.

TENOSYNOVITIS.   When tenosynovitis is the cause of pain, in
the absence of specific causative trauma, systemic disease must
be excluded. The cause of the tenosynovitis, however, may still
be repetitive, unnoticed minor trauma. When trauma is the cause,
treatment follows the principles outlined for the treatment of
tendinitis. But, to prevent adherence of the tendon to the sheath,
with resolution of the tenosynovitis, faradic stimulation of the
involved muscle of just sufficient intensity to move the tendon
in the sheath without pain is an important addition. Anodal
galvanism or phonophoresis using hydrocortisone (10% cream
— Griffin) accelerates the resolution of the condition.

INTRINSIC MUSCLES.   The intrinsic muscles are particularly
vulnerable to contusion, strain, fibrositis, and contracture from
lack of properly differentiated function. Specific muscle injuries
can scarcely be differentiated clinically, and the diagnosis usually
has to be made from the history and logical clinical inference.

Treatment.   Ice massage or vapor-coolant spray can readily be
applied to the most medially and most laterally situated intrinsic
muscles along the inner and outer borders of the foot. The treatment also is effective if applied over the dorsum of the foot in
the web areas when the deeper intrinsic muscles are involved.
In patients with chronic pathology of the intrinsic muscles, the
whole regimen of foot care (Chapter 7) must be followed. The
whirlpool or contrast baths are useful initially.

Bursitis, Bunions, and Ganglia

BURSITIS.   There are three common sites of bursitis in the
foot: (1) subcutaneous bursitis between the skin and the back
of the Achilles tendon at the top of the heel; (2) retrocalcaneal

bursitis between the Achilles tendon and the posterosuperior tubercle of the calcaneus; and (3) infracalcaneal bursitis beneath the inferior calcaneal tubercle, which is the area of maximum weight bearing. The signs of bursitis are clear in the first two cases, a tender, warm, localized fluctuant swelling being palpable at the anatomical site.

Signs of infracalcaneal bursitis are masked by the thick skin and subcutaneous tissues of the heel, and the diagnosis has to be inferential. The clue to the diagnosis is in the patient's shoe. Its heel insole is deeply hollowed out by wear, providing a concave trough in which the heel of the foot rests. The radiographic presence of a calcaneal spur in these patients is frequently and erroneously blamed as the pathological condition causing the symptoms. However, the spur remains present after successful treatment and the disappearance of the symptoms. It must also have preceded the onset of symptoms by months or years.

Treatment.   Each of these cases of bursal irritation is caused by shoe problems, and relief is achieved by appropriate shoe modifications. Local treatment by aspiration, injection of hydrocortisone, ultrasound — because of its property to increase the permeability of semipermeable membranes — and, if necessary, excision may also be done, but always with shoe modification.

In subcutaneous and infracalcaneal bursitis the heel of the foot may have to be protected from the posterior seam of the quarter. The quarter may have to be heightened or lowered, but usually the former. The heel stiffener may have to be removed. The heel may have to be heightened to relax the Achilles tendon.

In infracalcaneal bursitis the insole must be flattened and the weight bearing changed by sloping the heel with an anteroposterior wedge. There is a convenient commercial sponge rubber wedge heel that can be inserted into the shoe for this purpose; its upper surface is lined with leather. Unfortunately, it has a tendency to slip forward in the shoe, its posterior border becoming a cutting ledge over which the heel of the foot projects, thus aggravating rather than relieving the condition. Sponge-rubber doughnuts are contraindicated, as they also cause aggravating side-effects as the sole of the heel sinks into the hole of the doughnut. In recalcitrant bursitis the patient should be checked for the presence of gout or collagen vascular disease.

BUNIONS.   The acute pain of a bunion is due to acute bursitis, the bursa overlying the medial aspect of the first metatarsophalangeal joint in the big toe or, less commonly, the bursa overlying the lateral aspect of the fifth metatarsophalangeal joint. The former is associated with some degree of valgus deformity of the big toe, the latter with some degree of varus of the little toe. Both are caused by constant irritation of the joints and bursae by pressure from shoes that have the toes shaped too proximally, ill-designed toe stiffeners, or unfortunately placed stitching of the uppers.

Treatment.   Conservative treatment as outlined in Chapter 7 relieves the bursitis, but the cause in the shoe must be removed. Though the usual treatment is surgery, the problem will return sooner or later if the patient's shoes remain ill designed or ill fitting.

GANGLIA.   Ganglia were uncommon in the foot until the advent of surfing. Now, in communities where surfing is popular, they are commonplace (see Fig. 5-16).

If the surfer goes barefooted, he seems to be comfortable. I am aware of one instance in which sarcomatous changes were found in a surfer's ganglion, and this possibility should be kept in mind. Prior to the advent of surfing, I have seen ganglia on the dorsum of the foot only in relation to the mortise joint and the talonavicular joint.

Treatment. No treatment is required for ganglia, which are said to disappear within two years if left alone, unless they cause painful symptoms or interfere with function. In this case they can be ruptured, aspirated, or injected, though probably they are best excised.

Vascular Pain

The various causes of vascular pain have been discussed in Chapter 5, pages 106–108. Primarily, the treatment of pain from these causes is the treatment of the vascular disease, but there are physical therapy modalities that help to relieve the symptoms of pain in the feet.

ADJUNCTIVE PHYSICAL TREATMENT FOR VASCULAR PAIN. The different treatments are discussed briefly below:

1. *Reflex heating.* This can be achieved by body heating, avoiding direct application of heat to the affected limb. It probably works by central inhibition of the central nervous system, which produces indirect dilatation of the vessels of the extremities. A similar effect is thought to be produced by deep heat (shortwave) applied over the lumbar area of the back.
2. *Reflex chilling.* Circulatory improvement occurs with application of cold to the spine. Presumably this is also through an effect on the sympathetic nervous system.
3. *Coplanar short wave.* This treatment is given with one

pad electrode over the sole of the foot and the other in the small of the back. The improved circulation is probably produced by dilatation of the blood vessels of the muscles.

4. *Blocking of nerves*
   a. *Posterior tibial nerve* block, by a local anesthetic, enhances vasodilatation. The block is performed where the nerve courses around the medial malleolus.
   b. *Lumbar sympathetic block* involves introducing a local anesthetic about the lumbar sympathetic chain.
   c. *Caudal blocks* also work well and control pain of neuritic origin.

5. *Use of drugs*
   a. In early cases of arterial insufficiency *carbachol* or *methacholine* (*Mecholyl*) applied by iontophoresis over the dorsalis pedis area has a satisfactory effect on producing vasodilatation in the distal part of the foot.
   b. I have injected *papaverine* intraarterially in the early treatment of vascular deficiency in the foot. Pharmacologically this is a reasonable approach, but its effects are transient and its use should probably be limited to the first week of treatment.
   c. *Alcohol* by mouth produces vasodilatation, but its liberal use should not be recommended.

6. *Pneumatic machines.* Various pneumatic machines are manufactured and are of benefit in the presence of venous stasis or lymphatic edema.

7. *Faradic stimulation.* In that pumping of muscles is a prerequisite to efficient blood and lymph return to the circulation, faradic muscle stimulation can be of benefit only in a patient who has loss of vascular tone following, for instance, prolonged immobilization. This is applied with

the patient's lower limb elevated, thus allowing gravity to assist the circulation. For some reason, sufferers from seasonal vascular insufficiency in cold weather, especially in the hands and feet, are relieved by faradic stimulation exercise if it is started before cold weather sets in and is carried on through the winter.

8. *Exercises.* Buerger's exercise regimen, which is described on page 188, is of benefit to patients having arterial insufficiency in the lower extremities provided the adjunctive therapies are used in association with it. Not the least of these is the maintenance of a free exercise ambulation program within the limits of pain, which means within the capacity of the blood supply to the limb.

9. *Massage.* In the presence of edema resulting from stasis, massage is invaluable. This type of massage is a form of effleurage given centripetally, treatment starting in the thigh and progressing down the leg to the foot. It is a mechanical form of treatment which is assisted by elevation of the limb. Massage also "revitalizes" muscle by dispersing the waste products of its metabolism, which can only help in circulatory problems of all kinds. However, massage is contraindicated in arterial disease because it has the effect of dilating the skin vessels, which may create a reflex constriction of the deeper vessels to maintain circulatory equilibrium.

10. *Shoes.* In pseudointermittent claudication, raising the height of the heels of the shoes relieves the mechanical claudication symptoms (see Chapter 9).

11. *Supports.* Foot pain associated with varicose veins is partially relieved by the use of supporting hose. Better relief is obtained if every therapeutic approach mentioned above is enlisted.

Cramps

Although cramps are fundamentally due to circulatory problems, they are not necessarily symptoms of vascular disease. They
can be due to mechanical causes, arterial or venous disease,
neurological causes, and disordered metabolism. Restless legs at
night probably are precursors of cramps.

MECHANICAL CAUSES.   In the absence of vascular disease,
cramps in the feet may be due to internal muscle fatigue enhanced
by their physiopathological state resulting in poor flushing out
of catabolites. Overstrain or unaccustomed use of the extrinsic
muscles may also be to blame.
Treatment.   In these cases, treatment must be directed at the
cause, and any or all of the modalities mentioned previously to
correct muscle function may have to be used, especially faradic
foot baths, massage, supports, correction of heel height of shoes,
and muscle reconditioning by exercises. A most helpful treatment
that produces immediate relief of the pain of a cramped muscle
is the use of the vapor-coolant spray applied directly over the
cramped muscle. Quinine at night may prove a useful adjunct.

VASCULAR CAUSES.   Though cramps from vascular causes respond to the foregoing treatment modalities, these have no lasting
effect unless treatment of the underlying vascular condition is
undertaken. This is usually drug treatment and has to be adjusted
by experience. Some sort of combination of drugs, attacking from
all possible angles, is usually the most efficacious — that is, an
adrenergic blocking agent, with a drug acting on the smooth
muscle of the arterial tree and a drug having a central effect
together with gentle body warming for its reflex effect of vasodila-

tation on the peripheral vessels. Details of drug therapy fall into the province of specialists in peripheral vascular disease.

NEUROGENIC CAUSES.   Foot cramps may herald the onset of disease of the nervous system. They may be the presenting symptoms, for instance, of a disk prolapse, or perhaps a Morton's neuroma.

Treatment.   Treatment of cramps from neurogenic causes must be treatment of the cause, and no specific approach from a conservative point of view can be suggested.

TRIGGER POINTS.   The so-called trigger points may be the indirect cause of leg and foot cramps. Particularly, they can be found in the gastrocnemius-soleus group of muscles, often in the center of the calf. The cause of trigger points is not fully understood, but treatment of them is certainly efficacious. Gluteal trigger points may even cause cramping and pain in the foot and should be looked for on examination of the patient who has nebulous foot pain.

Janet Travell, M.D., states that myofascial trigger points mediate the pain of intermittent claudication in occlusive arterial disease of the legs. Treatment of them gives improvement, as measured by a treadlometer, walking, or toe-stand tests. It certainly seems that trigger areas in the calf muscles may themselves interfere with local blood flow by causing reflex vasospasm. Even in the presence of occlusive arterial disease, the myofascial component may be the major factor in maintaining a continuing pain cycle.

Treatment.   Trigger points are best treated by the use of vapor-coolant spray or ice massage with graduated passive stretching of the muscles in which they are situated.

Neuritic Pain

DIGITAL NEUROMA.   Excision relieves this condition so dramatically that other modalities of treatment need not be considered.

ASSOCIATED WITH VASCULAR DISEASE.   This type of foot pain improves with the treatment outlined for pain in vascular diseases in the foregoing sections.

NERVOUS SYSTEM DISEASE.   Diagnosis of the causative disease is prerequisite to treatment, which primarily is directed at the disease. Painful lower motor neuron neuritis is helped by hot packs, and if it is associated with muscle spasm, stretching as used in the Kenny treatment of poliomyelitis is helpful. With lower motor neuron paresis or paralysis, the foot must be properly supported to avoid contractures. Interrupted galvanic stimulation to denervated muscle, either resulting from lower motor neuron disease or peripheral nerve injury due to trauma or entrapment, is the only way to delay muscle atrophy. It must be given very frequently for short periods.

NEURITIC PAIN IN SCAR TISSUE.   Sometimes it seems that sensory nerve endings must become entrapped in scar tissue, either in superficial or in deep scars which may even be microscopic. When superficial, this can be treated by use of a vapor-coolant spray followed by pétrissage. Ultrasound, with its property of softening scar tissue, may be used with advantage. Local infiltration of local anesthetic and "needling" at the same time is often curative, providing the trauma from the needling is subsequently treated. Procaine can be introduced by iontophoresis and is effective; the positive electrode is active. Surgery may be required.

PRESSURE NEURITIS.   Two unusual clinical examples draw attention to the fact that pressure neuritis may be a cause of pain in the foot. In the first patient a new ski boot pressed over the ankle just behind the medial malleolus and produced pain and paresthesia under the anterior third of the sole of the foot. The other patient, when studying, supported his foot on a three-legged stool tilted backward so that the sole was flat on it but the heel was unsupported and the edge of the stool pressed across his instep. Treatment is to remove the cause. Recovery, although prolonged, is spontaneous.

Integument Pain

The problems of callosities, corns, and plantar warts have been dealt with elsewhere. Additional causes of discomfort, if not pain, are ingrowing toenails, epidermophytosis, hyperhidrosis, fungal infection of the nails, and blisters.

INGROWING TOENAILS.   Treatment of ingrowing toenails is prophylactic — that is, square cutting of the nails, which should be a universal practice. However, tight shoes from fashionable toe stiffeners, decorative brogues, or stitching may cause this problem in spite of good pedicare. Conservative therapy is limited to proper shoe fitting and pedicare.

TOENAILS.   Study of the toenails may not only provide the diagnosis of a foot pain problem but may also be rewarding in diagnosing systemic disease. Besides ingrowing toenails mentioned above, nail pain may be a feature of peripheral neuritis. Thickened nails from poor hygiene, especially in older people, may cause pain, and thickening of the nails may also occur with vascular disease. Following improper surgery for the removal of a toenail, pain may arise from nail regrowth which becomes ingrowing. A glomus tumor under the nail may be the cause of pain.

The nails become brittle with thyroid dysfunction, vitamin A deficiency, and in alcoholism, in which nail pain may be a feature.

There are characteristic nail changes which may be associated with pain that accompany anemia, sickle-cell disease, and fungus infections. Clubbing of the nails is associated with cardiac and chronic lung diseases, and parrot beaking with chronic dysentery.

Picked or torn toenails may indicate neurosis or other psychopathology and, of course, may also be a cause of pain. Paronychia may result from this or may be secondary to ingrowing nails or other local causes of infection, and is another cause of pain.

Fungal infections of the nails have been treated by application of aniline dyes and by exposure to ultraviolet light. Griseofulvin now is almost exclusively used.

EPIDERMOPHYTOSIS.   Without a doubt, copper iontophoresis is the most effective treatment of this condition. Copper is fungicidal. In the absence of proper foot hygiene, however, recurrences are common. Socks should be cotton so that they can be sterilized. Shoes should be treated with fungicidal powder.

HYPERHIDROSIS.   This condition of excessive sweating not only is unpleasant in itself but predisposes to epidermophytosis and the development of soft corns between the toes. Copper ionization alleviates the condition. Scrupulous foot hygiene and drying both with towels after washing and with powder during the day is necessary. Socks should be made of cotton. Nylon and wool aggravate the condition, as do rubber soled or plastic shoes.

BLISTERS.   Blisters occur as a result of irritation and rubbing from shoe defects and following the too early resumption of activity in the foot debilitated by disuse from any cause. They are painful, and if they become secondarily infected, they may be dangerous, especially if there is associated disease such as diabetes. Treatment is largely prophylactic in the prevention of too early return to function, attention to footwear (both shoes and socks), "toughening up" the "soft" foot, and general good foot hygiene.

7

Lower Extremity Injuries and Foot Pain

Morbidity occurs in the lower limbs and especially the feet from "modern" methods of treating fractures of the lower extremity and following surgical procedures performed on the lower extremities for any reason. One cannot divorce the foot from the ankle, the knee, and the hip or, for that matter, from the rest of the human body.

Following fractures or surgery in any part of the lower extremity and a successful local outcome of treatment, foot pain may supervene as a morbid and disabling result, even without direct involvement of the ankle and foot. This is pain of purely iatrogenic etiology and should be preventable. It is a sad reflection on medicine of our time that only in rehabilitative medicine is care of the whole patient stressed, and even then too often this is only lip service. Furthermore, it is a sad fact that the competent physiatrist is most often kept away from patients by their surgeons until morbid conditions are established, when it is often too late to do anything about them. It is gratifying to be able to reverse such complications, but how much better and easier it is to prevent them from occurring, and how much more economical in every way for the patient.

I make no apology, therefore, for the following detailed presentation of a program of treatment and management of a patient who has sustained fractures and other injuries to the lower limb. This program covers from the time of injury to the time of complete total physical restoration and is designed to minimize all morbid results following such an injury, the object of achieving normal feet being not the least part of the program. Unless a patient has a usable foot, it is of small benefit to him to have a good leg. So perhaps the whole program is really directed not toward ambulation per se, but toward the preservation of normal, painless feet on which to ambulate. The principles of the program are what matter; the local injury is truly incidental.

Prophylactic Treatment to Prevent Morbidity

Following any trauma, which includes fractures and surgery, to the lower extremity but which does not directly involve the foot, treatment should be instituted without delay to prevent morbid unnecessary changes occurring in those parts of the extremity not directly involved in the pathological process and especially the foot.

Depending on the severity and extent of the primary pathological conditions and the method used in their primary treatment, the areas that are available for prophylactic treatment vary. But the progressive treatment program which follows is a basic one, starting with massage and progressing through passive movement, assisted movement in bed, active assisted movement, early active movement unassisted, nonweight-bearing active movement, active movement with graduated resistance, initial weight bearing, and movement with weight bearing to the eventual achievement of free ambulation. The treatment program varies in timing and extent but not in principle, depending on the seat of the primary pathology. This program is used for a patient with a fractured hip.

MASSAGE.   Light massage (effleurage) is the initial modality of treatment. It is used to produce relaxation, relieve pain, reduce swelling, and enhance circulation. The therapist must remember, however, that in elderly people the use of massage must be limited to the least amount required to produce relaxation. In the aged, the reflex arc is easily tired, and prolonged massage produces the opposite of the desired effect. A few minutes of light stroking is sufficient to reduce protective spasm. Massage should progress from hip to foot.

PASSIVE MOVEMENT.   When the protective spasm and initial pain are overcome, movement is readily achieved with further impressive relief of pain. Note that the movement may be only a few degrees, and it is the determination of those few degrees that is basic to the skill of the therapist. As spasm is overcome, the first thing noted will be freedom of toe movement, and shortly after that the patient finds that he can move the ankle painlessly.

ASSISTED MOVEMENT IN BED.   At this point the therapist places a hand under the knee, which is gently raised and lowered each time the massaging hand passes over it (Fig. 7-1). As soon as it can be raised high enough painlessly, a pillow is placed beneath it; flexion and extension of the knee is then performed, the therapist supporting the ankle and assisting the movement from the ankle. It should take less than a quarter of an hour for the foot, ankle, and knee thus to be mobilized.

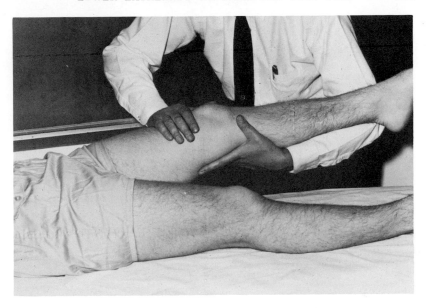

FIGURE 7-1.   The position the therapist adopts to support the knee during the early phase of administering assisted movement in bed while applying stroking massage.

ACTIVE ASSISTED MOVEMENT.   At this time the whole lower leg can be supported by the therapist, and pain-free movement of the hip can be started, each movement being slowly, carefully, and smoothly done. With evidence of either fatigue or the slightest pain, treatment is stopped, the limb is rested with the knee slightly flexed over a pillow (or with the bed slightly broken at the knee), and free movement of all the rest of the body is encouraged. The patient should be able to sit up in bed for short intervals throughout the day as soon as the period of traumatic shock is over (usually after 24 hours).

EARLY ACTIVE MOVEMENT.   In most cases the patient can be up in a chair (with skilled help to protect the hip) on the third day. The foot should be dependent and the patient encouraged throughout the day to move everything from, and including, the knee down to the toes.

NON-WEIGHT-BEARING ACTIVE MOVEMENT.   When early active movement is effortless, the patient is encouraged to stand on the unaffected leg and to begin gently swinging the injured leg. At this time, walking in a wading tank with water up to shoulder level is perfectly safe and most enjoyable for the patient. If a wading tank is not available, reambulation training is more tedious. It must not be started until there is perfect freedom of ankle and foot movement (including toe movement) and until, while sitting, perfectly coordinated swinging of both legs alter-

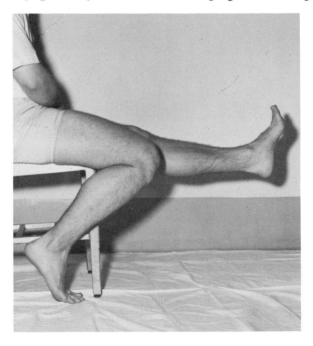

FIGURE 7-2.   The completion of the upward swing of the sitting leg-swinging exercise. Note the plantar flexion of the right foot (the toes would also be plantar flexed were the chair higher) and the right knee flexed and the dorsiflexion of the left ankle and toes, with the left knee fully extended.

nately and together is achieved without pain. This must be effort-less to the patient. The angle of swing is very small originally and is increased with increasing strength (Fig. 7-2). When the patient can hold the injured leg extended with the ankle and toes dorsiflexed for a count of three as well as he can the uninjured limb, and return to the flexed-knee position with the foot and toes plantar flexed, he is ready to progress to bicycling movements in air (Fig. 7-3). When these are achieved effortlessly, the patient stands between two chairs holding on to the backs and learns to swing the leg backward with the knee flexing and with the foot plantar flexing at the same time (Fig. 7-4). On swinging forward the knee should extend and the foot and toes should dorsiflex (Fig. 7-5). This simulates the normal coordinative movements of walking.

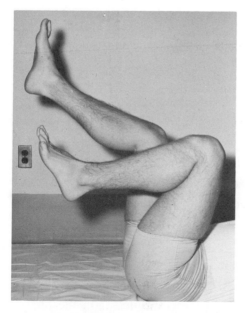

FIGURE 7-3. The free "bicycling" exercise which varies in extent depending on the degree of painless hip flexion that the patient can achieve.

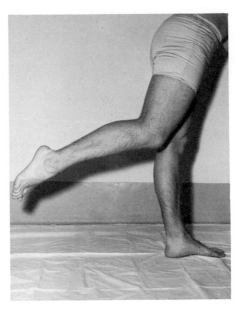

FIGURE 7-4. Backward phase of swinging the leg while standing. Note the plantar flexion of the ankle, the flexion of the toes, and the flexion of the knee on the right. For this exercise the patient should stand between two chairs for stability, but for clarity of illustration (Figs. 7-4 and 7-5), the model holds onto the back of one chair placed in front of him.

Next the patient sits with the knees flexed at slightly more than 90 degrees and the feet flat on the floor. The toes of each foot are raised and lowered from the floor while the heels remain on the floor. The knees are then further flexed and the foot movements repeated until the flexed position of the knees is such that it is impossible to raise the toes (Fig. 7-6). At this point the heels are each raised while the toes rest on the floor. This movement becomes increasingly limited as knee flexion is increased and stopped when no movement is possible (Fig. 7-7). Then these two exercises are combined with the knees at right angles over the edge of the chair — right toe, left toe, right heel, left heel, each tapping the ground in turn and performed rhythmically

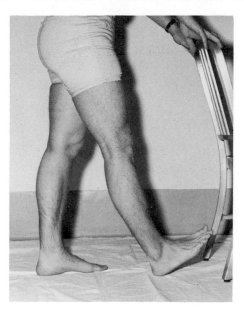

FIGURE 7-5. The forward phase of swinging the leg. The dorsiflexion of the ankle and toes and full extension of the knee on the right should be noted.

(Fig. 7-8). Between each exercise the patient is taught to sit with the ankles crossed and the feet inverted to rest on their lateral borders; in this position he should learn to claw the toes and arch the metatarsal heads (Fig. 7-9).

It should be noted that in none of the foregoing program is weight bearing exerted on the injured hip.

ACTIVE MOVEMENT WITH GRADUATED RESISTANCE. By the time the patient is proficient at the foregoing program — and he has been for some time completely independent about the house in transfer activities and *necessary* ambulation, using crutches, without bearing weight on the injured limb — he is ready to progress to a sliding-seat rowing machine. At first the sliding board is horizontal and the foot board is free. As strength returns,

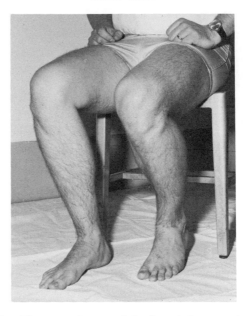

FIGURE 7-6.   The second stage of the first sitting exercise. The knees
are flexed to such a degree that raising the toes is no longer possible.
The heels are raised and lowered alternately.

the sliding board is raised from the horizontal and the foot board
is fixed in the position approaching horizontal which allows
maximum knee bend. Full extension of the knee must be ensured
by the therapist between each knee bend, thus assuring proper
function of the vastus medialis muscle, the stabilizing muscle of
the knee. Finally the patient progresses to exercises for specific
muscle groups of the hip of the injured leg using a rope, wall
pulley, and weights (Figs. 7-10 and 7-11).

INITIAL WEIGHT BEARING.   At this point, if the surgeon is
ready to permit weight bearing, the patient starts sitting with his
ankles cross-leg and the toes clawed, and he places his hands on
the chair seat and raises himself from it, keeping most of his
weight on the hands (Fig. 7-12). Each day he rises higher and

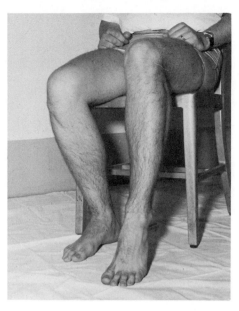

FIGURE 7-7.   The final stage of the first sitting exercise. The knees
are flexed to such a degree that the heels cannot reach the ground.

higher, taking more weight on the legs and the lateral aspect of
the feet and less on his hands, until he finally achieves the upright
position.

He now transfers his hands to the back of a chair placed in
front of him, again supporting much of his weight on his hands.
Taking the rest of his weight on the good leg, he uncrosses his
feet and stands on them, maintaining the weight on the outer
borders of the feet, and commences his first free standing exercise
— a simple knee-bending exercise through a few degrees only
(Fig. 7-13). These two exercises cannot be done by flat-footed
patients, unless their muscles are strong enough to prevent strain
of their plantar ligaments which would produce pain.

Next, standing on the good leg, the patient swings the other
leg back and forth, and then when the foot is falling from the

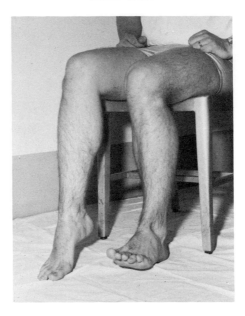

FIGURE 7-8.   The first two exercises in walking reeducation, combined. The toes and heels of both feet are raised and lowered alternately and at the same time.

front position, the heel is allowed to check its return by contact
with the ground (Fig. 7-14). Perfect coordination of this first
part of the natural walking step rapidly returns, with proper
power as well. When this is achieved without effort, as soon as
the heel checks the backswing, the body weight is thrown forward
so that the forefoot of the injured leg falls to the floor and the
heel of the good leg is raised from the floor. A rock to and fro is
then instituted without clawing the toes (Fig. 7-15). Then the
feet are reversed, the good one being in front and the injured
one behind, and rocking is continued. And so the patient progresses until the supporting chair back can be safely removed a
step and a half away from him. At this time he undertakes a step
and a half to and from the chair. The therapist continues his
supervision to ensure that the patient does heel-toe walking, keeps

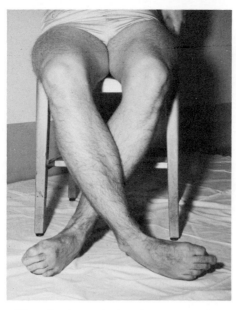

FIGURE 7-9.   The clawing of the feet exercise with the ankles
crossed.

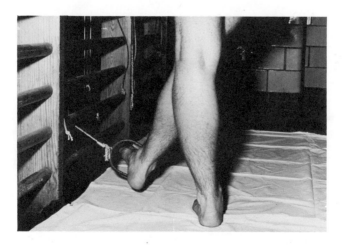

FIGURE 7-10.   Exercising the abductors of the hip using the wall
pulley. As the weight is increased, the exercise becomes an adductor
exercise as well.

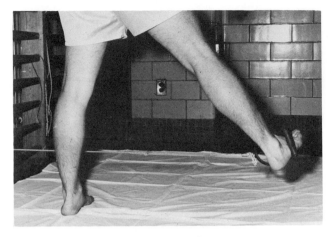

FIGURE 7-11.   The abductor exercise at its completion.

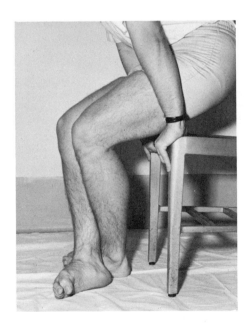

FIGURE 7-12.   Rising from the sitting position. The legs are still crossed at the ankle and the toes remain clawed. Most of the body weight is taken on the hands supported on the chair seat.

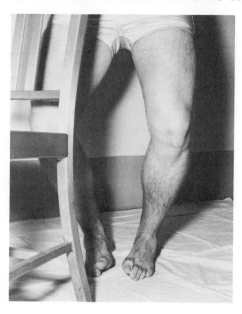

FIGURE 7-13. Simple knee bending, but with the weight of the body falling onto the outer borders of the feet.

his feet straight, and maintains his weight largely on the outer borders of the feet.

MOVEMENT WITH WEIGHT BEARING. The patient is now ready to resume full weight bearing. The progression should still be barefooted except when ambulation with a walker or in the parallel bars is undertaken. The therapist can guard against bad habits in ambulation only if the patient is barefooted. And bad habits may yet become a cause of foot pain. Practice walking, however, must be done in walking shoes — never slippers.

The patient stands with the weight of his body equally on the outer borders of both feet. The inner borders should be kept raised, but a little weight may be borne on them. The feet are parallel and about 4 inches apart. The knees are in full extension.

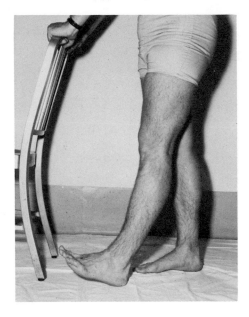

FIGURE 7-14. The patient takes the first quarter of a full step on
the left leg. The leg has been swinging and here, after the forward
swing, the return movement is checked when the heel is allowed to
hit the floor.

The body weight is thrown backward onto the heels, and then
forward gradually until most of the weight is on the head of the
fifth metatarsal bone (Fig. 7-16). The therapist must pay particular attention to see that the weight does not fall on the head
of the fourth metatarsal bone as well; if it does, splaying of the
foot occurs and metatarsalgia ensues.

A kind of circling movement is now performed, throwing the
weight from the fifth metatarsal head toward the first metatarsal
head while the heels are slightly raised from the floor (Fig. 7-17).
This exercise is then repeated, but with the toes turned inward and
the heels turned outward instead of the feet being parallel (Fig.
7-18). Then it is repeated again, this time with the heels together
and the toes turned outward. Flat-footed patients can do these

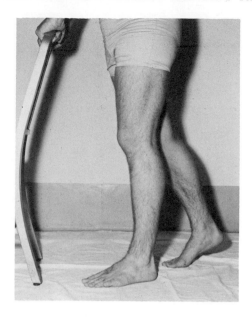

FIGURE 7-15.   The position adopted for rocking to and fro alternately on each leg. There must be no clawing of the toes of either foot.

exercises only if their muscle strength is sufficient to prevent strain on the plantar ligaments, which would produce pain. Raising and lowering the inner sides of the feet with the toes clawed (Fig. 7-19) is then followed by standing on the heels and raising the toes (Fig. 7-20).

The exercise that follows is that of knee bending, first with the feet parallel and the knees together, and then with the heels together and the toes and knees apart but maintaining the long axis of the thigh parallel to the long axis of the foot (Figs. 7-21 and 7-22). This exercise must not be done in a slovenly manner or too quickly. The heels are raised and the knees fully extended. Then knee bending is slowly performed, flexion of the knee being equal on both sides. Squatting, which should aim to get down to the heels, must be maintained for a slow count of three,

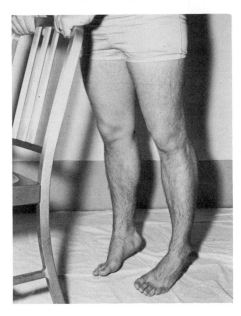

FIGURE 7-16.   Showing the first position for tiptoe exercise. Body weight is maintained on the outer borders of the feet. The feet are kept parallel and about 4 inches apart. The knees are in full extension. The body weight is carefully thrown forward until most of the weight is on the heads of the fifth metatarsals, as shown.

and the return should be made to tiptoe with the knees fully extended before resting. As soon as the patient has learned this routine, he should perform it on his own three times a day.

FREE AMBULATION.   When free ambulation is achieved without a limp, the patient should be encouraged consciously to be sure that he walks with heels and toes parallel (see Fig. 3-2), and to stand with the toes slightly turned in and the knees braced in full extension. He must also consciously maintain the heel-toe gait. If the patient is nervous or weak, he should be encouraged to use Canadian canes — two, not one. There is no failure or shame in this, and it gives him added stability and safety.

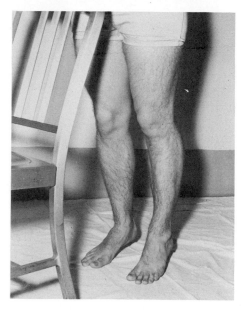

FIGURE 7-17.   Continuing the exercise shown in Figure 7-16, the
weight is transferred smoothly from the fifth metatarsal head toward
the first metatarsal head in a "circling" motion.

The entire program of treatment just described should be
followed for patients with hip fractures and modified when the
primary pathology is elsewhere in the lower limb.

Specific Injuries

IMPACTED FRACTURE OF NECK OF FEMUR.   Impacted fractures of the neck of the femur really require no surgical treatment,
and if physical therapy is started from the beginning, little, if any,
disability should ensue when healing is complete. It is possible,
even probable, that more people die from treatment by immobilization in these cases than from the injury itself. However, if
surgeons feel safer because they put pins in these fractures, let

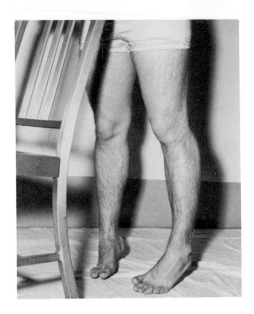

FIGURE 7-18. Same exercise illustrated in Figure 7-16 but with the toes turned inward and the heels turned outward.

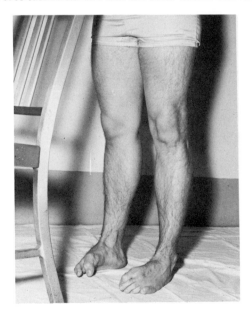

FIGURE 7-19. The patient raises the inner aspect of the feet while the toes perform the clawing exercise.

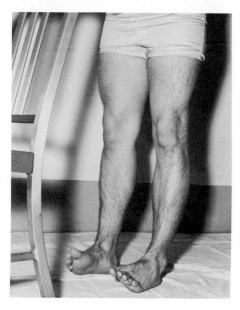

FIGURE 7-20.   The exercise in which the patient stands on his heels. The inner borders of the feet must be raised more than the outer borders.

them put them in. But just because they feel safe about the fracture, let them not then forget the patient. Already the surgery has contributed some morbidity, and recovery is proportionately slower. When patients with these injuries are treated by trained physical therapists, using massage and mobilization techniques, they do remarkably well.

HIP JOINT DISLOCATION.   The program of physical treatment following dislocation of the hip joint is the same as that for an impacted fracture both prior to the resumption of weight bearing and after ambulation is permitted by the surgeon. It is very probable that aseptic necrosis of the head of the femur would occur less frequently if the whole limb were always treated according to physiological principles.

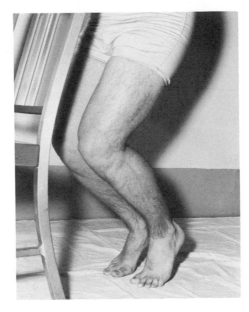

FIGURE 7-21.   Heel raising and knee bending with the heels together
and knees directly in line with the feet, which are kept parallel.

NONIMPACTED FRACTURES OF NECK OF FEMUR. These
fractures require internal fixation of one kind or another, but
even though there is a surgical wound to heal, there need be and
should be no delay in putting the patient on the treatment program outlined above. It is customary for the surgeon not to allow
full weight bearing for at least 6 months following these fractures.
The program outlined above has the patient ready for ambulation
in about 2 months; this satisfactory physical state simply has to
be maintained by the patient, preferably supervised from time
to time by the therapist to ensure no backsliding by the patient
while awaiting the go-ahead from the surgeon.

If a replacement prosthesis is used by the surgeon, there is no
change in the program except that free ambulation is usually
permitted as soon as the training program is completed. In these

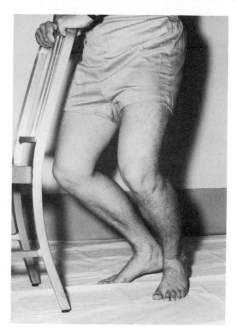

FIGURE 7-22.   Same exercise as in Figure 7-21, with the toes and knees apart but maintaining the long axis of the thigh parallel with the long axis of the foot.

cases, the program may be accelerated, but the therapist must avoid external rotation and adduction movements in the first 4 weeks of treatment.

INTERTROCHANTERIC AND SUBTROCHANTERIC FRACTURES OF FEMUR.   Internal fixation of these fractures usually requires a longer surgical procedure and the operative shock is correspondingly prolonged. The initiation of the initial phase of the treatment program need not be delayed, but the early progress is slower. However, healing is usually faster than with a femoral neck fracture, and free ambulation is usually permitted in 4 months. Thus, the maintenance period following physiological recovery is shortened and is less tedious to patient and therapist.

SHAFT FRACTURES OF FEMUR. The program of physical treatment in these cases depends on whether the treatment of the fracture is by internal fixation or by the use of balanced skeletal traction and a spica cast, each phase of which takes about 6 to 8 weeks or about 4 months in all. If internal fixation is used, there need be no modification of the program already described, but the return to free ambulation is delayed by some surgeons for as much as a year. The treatment by traction followed by a cast, however, complicates the therapist's job, sometimes to a heart-breaking degree.

It is in balanced traction that many foot problems start, and if the foot is not treated from the beginning, the morbid changes that result may be so severe by the time the surgeon is satisfied that the fracture has healed that full correction by physical treatment is impossible.

First, the cradling sling of the Pearson attachment which supports the lower leg is frequently applied so that its lower edge cuts across the Achilles tendon. The foot, often unsupported, adds weight to the forces already damaging this vital structure. Furthermore, if the forefoot is allowed to drop forward, both the Achilles tendon and the plantar fascia shorten rapidly, and an iatrogenic pes cavus develops. These things must be promptly corrected. Foot massage and movement must be instituted from the day the traction apparatus is applied. Ankle movements must also be prescribed. The lower leg can be massaged and relaxed movement given to the knee.

For some reason, the insertion of a pin through the femoral condyles or through the usual area behind the tibial tuberosity is often the precursor of a "frozen" knee. This condition, once established, is most recalcitrant to treatment, but I believe it is preventable by the use of relaxed movements to the knee from the outset and by the use of faradic muscle stimulation and massage to the thigh muscles from the start. Certainly, a "frozen" knee compounds the problems of the foot in these cases. While giving treatment movement to the knee the therapist has to maintain the traction forces, as the Pearson attachment has to be loosened to give the treatment. The Pearson attachment has to be reattached to its weight before the therapist removes his manual traction at the knee after the therapy session. The patella must be kept mobile in every range of its joint-play movements. The occurrence of muscle spasm during treatment is easily appreciated by the therapist and warns him to stop what he is doing before the patient experiences pain. During pain-free treatment no harm can come to the fracture. The maintenance of activity as normal physiologically as possible can only promote the healing process.

With these modifications, the treatment program should follow that outlined at the beginning of the chapter. To consolidate healing and promote an early safe return to function, the program should continue as detailed when the traction is removed. However, the patient is usually put into a spica at this point. Quite obviously, this not only undoes all the good that therapy has achieved but it starts off a whole new train of morbid conditions which are probably worse than if nothing had been done to the patient while he was in traction. The foot on the injured side usually is now completely neglected, the knee which has been kept mobile becomes stiff, as does the hip, the muscles all will atrophy, and even the good leg is going to have its function impaired to some degree. Even if ambulation in the spica is encouraged — an extremely difficult physical feat even for an athletic young man — the movement he can perform is unnatural and is limited to that which is possible from the knee down. At least, isometric exercises can be done for the quadriceps of both legs, the uninjured lower leg maintained in as normal state as possible, and both feet can and must be cared for according to the principles of good physical treatment. The upper half of the body can also have its normal physiological state maintained.

TIBIAL PLATEAU FRACTURES.   Treatment of fractures of the tibial plateau may require surgical intervention; if so, it may be undertaken immediately after injury or after healing of the fracture, depending on the individual preference of the surgeon. My experience in treating these fractures using a plaster leg-length back splint, with the knee resting in its most comfortable position, has been good. This method of treatment for the fracture allows early physical therapy by massage and mobilization following the usual principles, and the foot and ankle can be cared for from the start. Even if the leg is put in plaster, if the cast is bivalved the foot and ankle can readily be cared for from the onset of the fracture treatment. Nor is there any reason why the patella should not be kept mobile all the time to lessen morbid knee changes which delay the early return of function of the whole extremity.

FRACTURES OF THE PATELLA.   As surgical removal of a fragment (or fragments) of bone is the usual treatment for this injury, and as the use of a plaster cast, for some reason, is almost routine following orthopedic surgical procedures, the same principles of treatment designed to assist a patient's return to ambulatory independence must be followed.

Most transverse fractures heal readily if the principles of massage and movement are followed. The leg, which is not in a cast, is kept in elevation and extension. The swelling is overcome by gravity and massage. The bone fragments are approximated by strapping applied in a horseshoe manner around the lower fragment, and as the swelling disappears, the strapping is reinforced daily, if necessary with added upward tension in the new application maintaining the approximation of the bone fragments. In this instance the use of elastoplast is preferable to adhesive tape. The slight elasticity maintains apposition of bone at the fracture site as the excess synovial fluid and edema are absorbed.

The muscles of the upper and lower leg and the feet are maintained in their physiological state. Relaxed knee movements are normally possible within 4 weeks, and the morbid complications of the injury are kept to a minimum. Weight bearing can usually be resumed without protection in 8 weeks. This conservative treatment was advocated by Sir Robert Jones in his book *Injuries to Joints*.

OTHER PROCEDURES ABOUT THE KNEE.   Following meniscectomy or surgical repair of a ruptured quadriceps tendon or patella ligament, patients should be treated using these same principles. If, following abdominal surgery, surgeons consider it safe to use very early ambulation in their postoperative care, then it is surely as safe if not safer to use the methods of treatment advocated here to prevent morbid complications following what amounts to soft tissue surgery in the extremities. The musculature of the abdomen is seldom in as viable and normal a state as is that of the lower extremities. Physical restoration following rupture and repair of any of the ligaments of the knee joint also should follow the same principles.

FRACTURES OF THE TIBIA AND FIBULA.   It is hoped that the knee-jointed long leg plaster recently advocated by Dr. Verne Nichol will receive ready acceptance and thus prevent morbid knee complications following fractures now treated by immobilization in a long leg plaster. Meanwhile, one must still expect morbid changes in the foot and ankle following routine forms of treatment. They can be largely avoided if physical therapy is instituted just as soon as the fracture (or fractures) has become adequately "sticky," usually in about 4 weeks. Morbidity can also be lessened if care is taken to maintain the foot in plaster without any plantar flexion and if the plaster incorporates a platform to support the toes; each of the toes should always be visible as far proximally as the proximal aspects of all the metatarsopha-langeal joints, thus allowing free movement of all the digits.

Pain in the "ankle" from joint dysfunction in the subtalar joint is almost inevitable after immobilization of any part of the leg in plaster. It responds readily to the restoration of normal joint play by joint manipulation. Pain in the foot is also invariably present, and this too largely arises from joint dysfunction in the other tarsal joints and is readily relieved by manipulation followed by reeducation, as outlined above.

The lower third of the tibia is subject to stress fractures, which is particularly to be remembered when dealing with recruits in the armed services. Altered sound conduction of bone, heard through the stethoscope, is a valuable sign of long-bone fracture which could be used to advantage by army doctors.

RUPTURE OF THE ACHILLES TENDON.   This condition has to be treated in plaster with the foot initially in plantar flexion, but frequent plaster changes lessening the angle of plantar flexion each time minimize the foot complications. Following treatment for this condition, joint dysfunction in the mortise joint is an added complication, but this also responds to manipulative therapy. As the Achilles tendon (and plantaris muscle) is an integral part of the musculature of the entire leg — not just the lower leg — restorative treatment has to be directed at the whole limb and not just the ankle region.

RUPTURE OF THE TIBIAL COLLATERAL (DELTOID) OR FIBU-LAR COLLATERAL LIGAMENT.   Ruptured ligaments are probably more serious injuries than fractures around the ankle, but the principles of restorative treatment are the same. The performance of surgery for repair or internal fixation of any of these conditions in no way alters their after-treatment.

FRACTURES OF THE TALUS. This is one of the fractures which early radiological examination may not reveal. Fat in the blood aspirated from a hematoma in the injured area, especially in the region of the sinus tarsi, should alert one to the presence of a fracture of the talus. Aseptic necrosis is said to be a common complication of a fractured talus. There are no special features in the approach to treatment beyond the principles already outlined.

FRACTURES OF THE CALCANEUS. This bone is subject to stress fracture, a fact especially to be remembered by doctors who are responsible for the care of army recruits. Often a calcaneal fracture is difficult to detect radiographically unless one remembers that the angle subtended by the horizontal axes of the talus and calcaneus is normally 35 degrees. Anything less than that is very suggestive of a calcaneal fracture (Fig. 5-2). The calcaneus is usually a "mushy mess" when it is fractured, and the subtalar joint is often irreversibly injured, eventually necessitating subtalar fusion. But whether or not surgery is required, the postfracture treatment follows the same principles as above.

FRACTURES OF THE METATARSAL BONES. Except that the distal shafts of the metatarsal bones may be the site of stress fractures (Fig. 5-1) (march fractures), a fact again specially to be remembered in service-training camps, there is nothing in particular to add regarding the prophylactic treatment program to prevent subsequent foot pain. However, most metatarsal fractures are readily treated by wearing a well-fitting shoe 24 hours a day, with no weight bearing, until healing takes place. If the foot is properly treated daily as well, very little disability should result, though a metatarsal-head support (see Chapter 8) may be required in spite of a good restoration treatment program before permanent comfort is obtained.

FRACTURES OF THE PHALANGES.   Strapping of the injured toe to an adjacent uninjured toe is usually adequate to allow for healing of the fracture. A rocker bottom on the shoe of the involved foot (see Chapter 10) should allow necessary but restricted ambulation during the healing process. Except for the need to mobilize the metatarsal heads and the metatarsophalangeal joints after healing no further treatment is normally required to assure a pain-free foot.

Foot pain following fractures of any of the bones of the feet is often proportional to the amount of bleeding and edema that is associated with the initial trauma besides the length of time of immobilization employed. The fascia, and especially the plantar fascia, readily contracts with immobilization; this is particularly true if the foot is immobilized with any undue degree of dropping of the forefoot. Usually, the intrinsic muscles, even before a fracture, at best are in a pathophysiological state, and the more the bleeding and edema, the more the balance shifts from the physiological to the pathological side; also, the longer the disuse, the further still will the shift be. Disuse will produce atrophy and fibrosis of these muscles, even further disturbing their already poor function, and too early return to weight bearing will compound these insults and injuries. Shoe adaptations or even special shoes (see Chapter 11) may be a vital part of physical restoration in these patients. If the foot is immobilized, splayed, or carelessly positioned in any position of stress, the ligaments of the multiple joints may stretch. If there is cramping of the foot in the immobilization device, these ligaments may unduly contract. Thus every anatomical structure in the foot may require very special attention if foot pain is not to be a most disabling sequel to any foot injury.

Though the reader may find himself at a loss to understand why this prolonged section on the treatment of fractures of the lower extremity is included in a book on foot pain, on reflection he will realize that foot pain with subsequent disability is a common complication of leg fractures, and the chapter is directed at the subject of prophylaxis against the occurrence of foot pain by the use of intelligent and reasoned programs of physical therapy.

8

Exercise Therapy

Exercise therapy, of the usual modalities of physical treatment, is prescribed, usually empirically, for most painful musculoskeletal conditions. Most often the prescriber has little, if any, idea how to carry out his suggested program and leaves the details to a trained physical therapist if the patient is lucky or, if less fortunate, to anyone — office nurse, parent, or physical education "specialist" or teacher — who has to interpret as best he or she may from printed illustrations of what the prescriber intends.

Before exercise therapy is discussed, it is well to review the principles that are inherent in any form of physical treatment.

Principles of Physical Therapy

It should first be recognized that modalities of physical therapy, for the most part, never cure anyone of anything. The exceptions are certain uses of ultraviolet light when it is bactericidal, iontophoresis of heavy metals (copper) which is fungicidal and is especially useful in the eradication of epidermophytosis of the feet (athlete's foot), and joint manipulation — as described by the author — which reverses joint dysfunction and restores joint play, thus relieving pain and restoring function.

For the rest, physical therapy modalities are used: (1) to change the climate in and around a pathological process to promote healing; (2) to maintain normal physiological processes in structures not directly involved in the pathological process; (3) to prevent the establishment of morbid changes in structures not involved directly in the primary pathological process; and (4) to restore function that may be lost as a result of the healing of a pathological process. If the first three principles are adhered to, less difficulty arises in the restoration phase exemplified by the fourth principle.

In the treatment of pathological conditions arising in the musculoskeletal system, and particularly in treating those which result from trauma, the first two principles of treatment are to rest from function (not just rest) that structure which is directly involved in the pathological process producing the symptoms, while maintaining everything else in as normal a state as possible.

In dealing with joint pathology — that is, any pathological condition involving the bone adjacent to the articular cartilage, the hyaline articular cartilage itself, the synovial capsule, or the supporting ligaments — the joint must be rested from function while the muscles are maintained in as normal a physiological state as possible.

In dealing with joints, rest from function does not mean immobilization except in the rarest circumstances, and the only condition I can think of that requires absolute immobilization is acute hematogenous osteomyelitis. For other pathological conditions any movement is better than no movement. The degree of permitted movement is that which can be performed passively and painlessly. The trained physical therapist recognizes this in the prescription ordering "passive range of movement within the limit of pain." Most (orthopedic) surgeons are frightened by this concept because it is difficult for them to visualize 1 degree of movement of anything, nor can any but a well-trained therapist carry out such a prescription safely. To the average person anything less than say 10 degrees is not movement; but it is, and is very important in the prevention of morbidity. Add to this prescription an initial word "graduated" and the trained therapist knows how and when safely to increase the dose of movement both qualitatively and quantitatively. This is not treatment by manipulation.

In dealing with joints, maintenance of normal physiology in those structures unaffected primarily by the pathological process means treating the muscles, fascia, and skin, but especially the muscles. This means that the muscles must be kept moving without joint function and invokes the use of isometric exercises. If a patient is unable to perform them, they can be carried out by using the faradic current. To simulate normal physiological activity, hand-surged faradic current is best. The most important part of the treatment is that the surging contraction phase be cycled to allow the refractory period and relaxation period to be completed. Muscle fatigue must be avoided, and this requires a trained therapist to be in attendance. Frequent short sessions of treatment are obviously better than a single prolonged one. To attach a patient to a machine which surges current under metronomic control is unphysiological and may be harmful. If the patient is able to do isometric exercises, he must learn to do them frequently and properly throughout his waking hours and must be taught the physiological cycle of muscle action.

Relaxation before the performance of any exercise program enhances the efficiency of the prescription, and for this purpose heat may be prescribed. It must be recognized, however, that heat, while increasing the blood flow, in the presence of traumatic pathology only increases the blood flow *to* the injured part and not away from it. Heat alone in these circumstances produces and increases congestion. It is the pumping action of muscle that increases the blood flow and, for that matter, the lymph drainage *away* from the injured part. This may be enhanced by antigravity positioning of the injured part. Also, to assist the venous and lymph return, massage is obviously of value and should be used. Massage also maintains the normalcy of the integument of the part. In the presence of severe local pain such as arises from an injured ligament or bruised periosteum, and in the presence of localized and painful swelling, the use of anodal (or medical) galvanism is difficult to improve upon. In addition to its effect of increasing the threshold of the sensory nerve endings, producing an appreciable anesthetic effect, anodal galvanism tends to lessen swelling of any kind, presumably by an iontophoretic effect on the salt content of the tissue or body fluid. If the swelling is due to blood, the addition of Wydase (a hyaluronidase preparation) to the electrolyte fluid at the anode makes the tissue fluid less viscous and promotes its dispersal or absorption.

Specific Programs

Exercise therapy is (or should be) used to do something primarily to muscles and only secondarily to joints. For exercise therapy to be successful, the joints upon which the muscles act must be free to move. In the presence of joint disease or deformity, exercise therapy not only is almost certain to fail but is more likely under such circumstances to aggravate the pathological condition causing the pain, which the therapy is prescribed to relieve.

Before active exercise therapy is prescribed, any active pathological process must be quiescent. Any degree of joint dysfunction must be treated and normal joint play restored before the muscles can begin to be trained to resume their normal function. It can be stated justifiably that all painful feet have joint dysfunction in virtually all their joints, whatever the primary underlying pathology may have been. In shoe-wearing people widespread joint dysfunction can be demonstrated even in "normal" feet. Joint manipulation, then, must almost always precede exercise therapy in the feet.

In shoe-wearing people it is, to all intents and purposes, a sine qua non that at least the intrinsic muscles of the feet demonstrate alienation — that is, they have lost their ability to respond to the neuromuscular control and cannot perform their specific action — and that they are all in a pathophysiological state. It is impossible to reeducate alienated muscles by active exercise, or even by assisted active exercise. It may therefore be necessary initially to overcome this situation by the use of faradic stimulation. In the foot this is achieved by the use of faradic foot baths.

FARADIC FOOT BATHS.   The foot is placed in a bath of warm water with the heel resting on a flat electrode. The water should be deep enough to reach the level of the malleoli. A moving electrode is then placed in the water, and while the current is surged (preferably manually by the therapist), the electrode is moved around the foot. Surging may be achieved by moving the electrode smoothly and rhythmically toward and away from the foot. The important thing is that every muscle in the foot should be exposed to stimulation, and this can be done only if the electrode is kept moving about in the bath until treatment has been administered in every position from the external malleolus around to the internal malleolus along the outer border of the foot, along the inner border of the foot, and over the whole dorsum of the foot.

MASSAGE. Following a faradic foot bath the whole foot, and indeed the whole lower leg, should be massaged. It is helpful to use a lubricant cream containing a rubefacient in massaging the foot — for example, Lembrose (Wyeth) which contains methacholine chloride. The massage to the foot is a firm but not heavy effleurage. The plantar aspect of the foot is massaged largely by using the thenar eminence of the hand, which snugly fits the plantar contours of the foot. The dorsal aspect of the foot is massaged largely by use of the thumb. It is important not to leave out the compartments behind the malleoli and in front of the Achilles tendon, where gentle kneading with the thumb and fingers is easily performed. The lower leg is then subjected to massage in the usual whole-handed manner. For the lower leg, talcum powder or some other lubricant is used.

The patient is ready for exercise therapy usually within 10 to 14 days. The time is judged from the clinical response, the return of suppleness and diminished tenderness. Assisted exercise is prescribed. This is better considered as manual muscle training.

MANUAL MUSCLE TRAINING. The physical therapist places the ball of his thumb on the sole of the foot so that it fits exactly into the concavity formed by the heads of the metatarsal bones; if the hand is too far forward, it will press on the heads of the metatarsals and cause pain. The patient is encouraged to claw with his toes. The foot is maintained in dorsiflexion by the therapist (Fig. 8-1). An arch is thus formed by the therapist while the patient's muscles are taught to maintain it. Clawing of the toes brings the lumbricals into effective action. When the patient has learned this rather simple function, the therapist changes his stabilizing grip and arches the metatarsal heads from the dorsal aspect of the foot, and the patient then learns to claw the toes

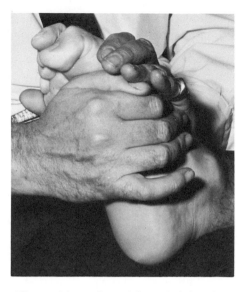

FIGURE 8-1. The position adopted for administering assisted exercises after mobilizing the metatarsal heads for metatarsalgia. The patient claws the toes over the therapist's hand, which supports the metatarsals just proximal to the metatarsal heads.

and dorsiflex the ankle himself at the same time (Figs. 8-2 and 8-3).

ACTIVE EXERCISE. Having become proficient at this, the patient no longer needs the assistance of the therapist and can progress to a device-assisted exercise using a Patterson's foot board (Fig. 8-4). The therapist teaches the patient to regulate the resistance of the foot board, and then this part of the program can be performed at home.

From this the patient progresses to learning how to pick up a large marble, then a golf ball, and finally a tennis ball with the foot. The ball is placed on the floor well behind the ball of the foot. The foot is then slowly pulled backward, rolling the ball beneath it, while the patient claws down on it until he is able to clasp

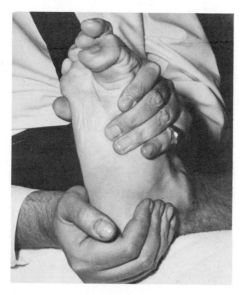

FIGURE 8-2. Adding further movement and resistance to the exercise illustrated in Figure 8-1. Now the clawing of the toes is assisted from above by the therapist's left hand, which also resists dorsiflexion at the ankle.

it and pick it up. The completion of this exercise is illustrated in Figures 8-5 and 8-6. In positioning to perform this exercise, the extensor muscles are brought into play, together with the abductors of the big and little toes, and the extrinsic muscles which are used to stabilize the foot during the grasping process.

FREE EXERCISE. Free exercises are then initiated to maintain the suppleness of the foot, its newly achieved dexterity, and the more normal physiological function of the muscles. Many devices have been designed to assist a patient in this, but the best I have come across is that which passes under the trade name of Vita-Ped (formerly Vimulator). This device is simple, effective, and inexpensive. It consists of a wooden frame over which is stretched a rubberized cover. Within the framework, strategically placed,

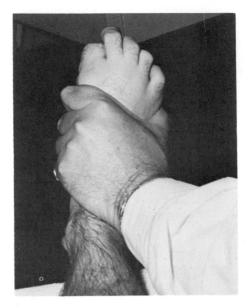

FIGURE 8-3.   Exercise shown in Figure 8-2 but from the dorsal
aspect of the foot.

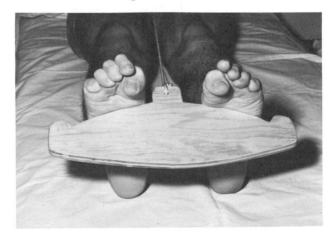

FIGURE 8-4.   The Patterson foot board which is made of wood and
is 9½ by 5 by 1 inches in size. The patient, whose knees are fully extended, holds the cord tightly and pulls enough to maintain the
ankles in full dorsiflexion. The curved edges of the board are placed
behind the metatarsal heads, and the metatarsophalangeal joints are
flexed over them and the toes are clawed.

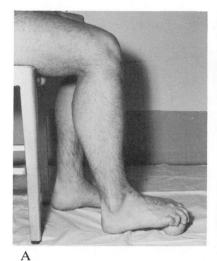
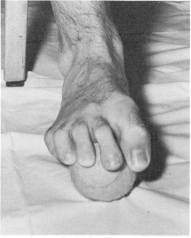

A   B

FIGURE 8-5.   The grip required to pick up a tennis ball with the foot. A. The lateral view. B. The front view. The ball has been rolled from under the instep forward to the toes.

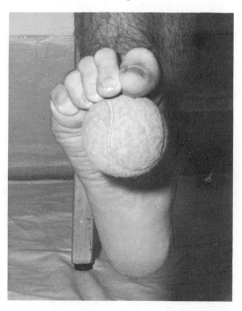

FIGURE 8-6.   The ball shown in Figure 8-5 has been successfully picked up.

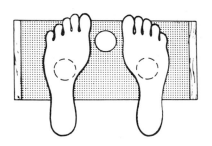

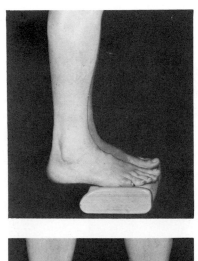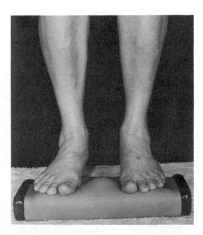

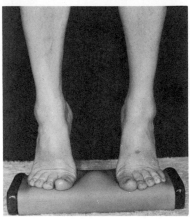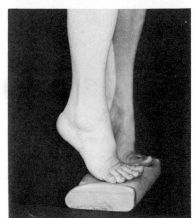

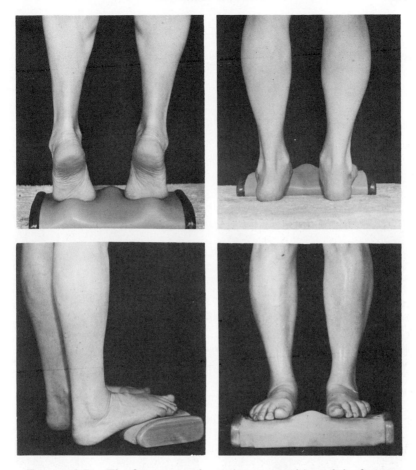

FIGURE 8-7. The first group of exercises and position of the feet on the Vita-Ped.

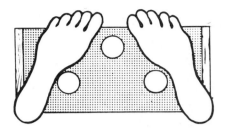

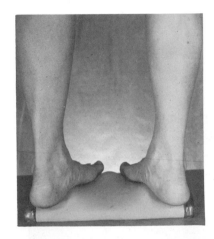

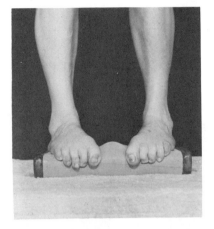

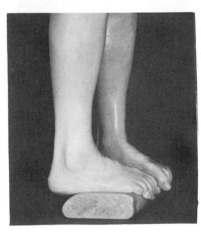

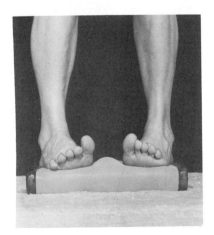

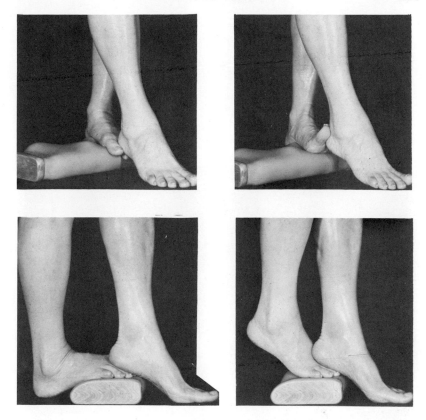

FIGURE 8-8. The second group of exercises and position of the feet on the Vita-Ped.

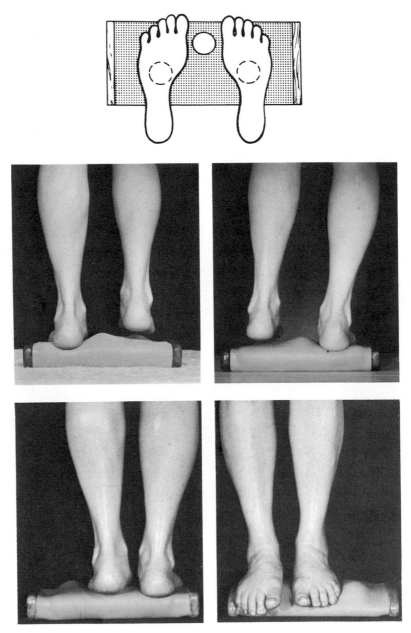

FIGURE 8-9.   The third group of exercises and position of the feet
on the Vita-Ped.

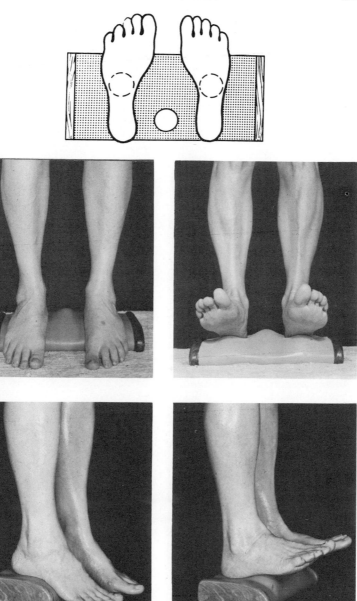

FIGURE 8-10.   The fourth group of exercises and position of the feet
on the Vita-Ped.

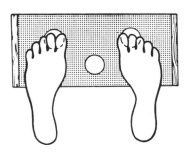

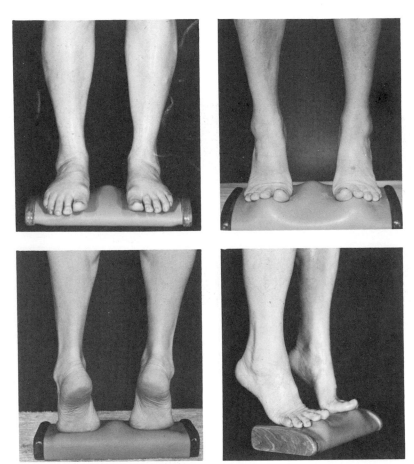

FIGURE 8-11. The fifth group of exercises and position of the feet on the Vita-Ped.

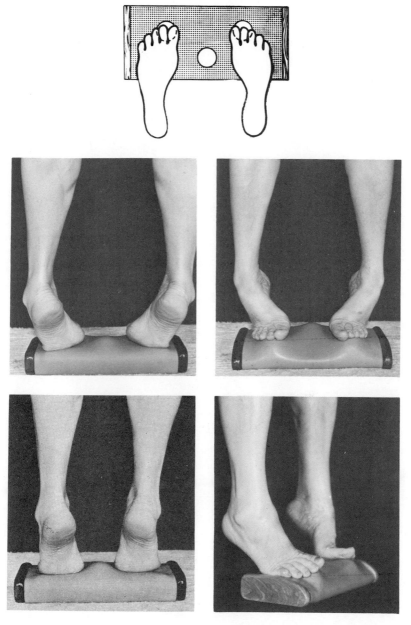

FIGURE 8-12. The sixth group of exercises and position of the feet on the Vita-Ped.

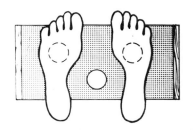

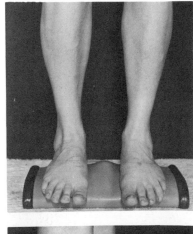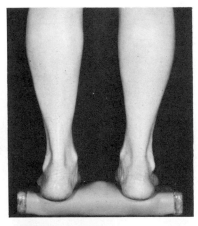

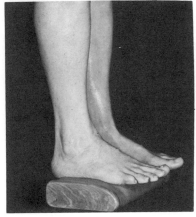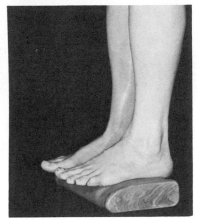

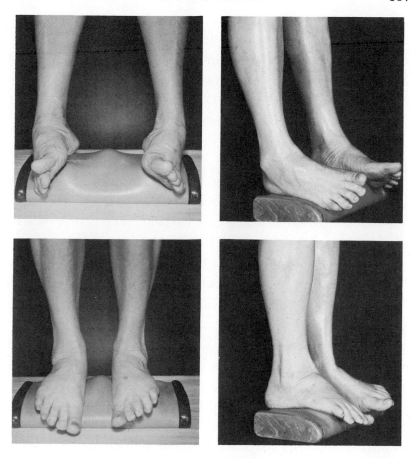

FIGURE 8-13.   The seventh group of exercises and position of the feet on the Vita-Ped.

are three rubber balls about the size of tennis balls. The placement of the feet on and around the balls determines the nature of muscle and joint activity in the user's feet. Figures 8-7 through 8-13 show the seven exercises and the position of the feet for each exercise. If all these suggested exercises are performed, with the feet placed around the balls as shown, all the muscles and joints in the feet are brought into activity.

REMEDIAL EXERCISES.   For remedial purposes, one cannot do better than to follow the exercise regimen of the ballet dancer. For such a program there can be none better than that devised by Raoul Gelabert, L.P.T.

The relief of foot pain cannot be expected by any sort of treatment if the principles of physical therapy are ignored. It cannot be stressed too strongly that if freedom from pain is to be achieved, rest from function during the healing and restorative phases of treatment is imperative. The time to resume function is when muscles are judged "good" on manual muscle testing and when that testing is achieved without pain. One cannot expect to overcome long-standing foot deformities, and the pain arising from them, by these methods, nor can any of these measures be of lasting value to a patient who persists in wearing or resumes wearing shoes into which he must cram his feet.

BUERGER'S EXERCISES.   Exercise regimens in the treatment of pain in the feet arising from vascular causes are of little use alone, but when used in conjunction with the absolute cessation of smoking and with the administration of various vasodilating drugs, with or without sympathectomy, they may help to delay the progression of pathological changes and therefore merit attention. In Buerger's exercises the patient's legs are first elevated on three pillows until they are ischemic (judged by pallor or the development of pain). He then sits on the edge of the bed with the legs hanging down until they first become hyperemic and then the hyperemia disappears. This is followed by a rest period in the horizontal supine position for a few minutes, after which the cycle is repeated. The duration of the exercise is from ½ to 1 hour and should be repeated three or four times a day. Timing of each phase of the cycle depends on how long it takes for ischemia to develop in the leg-up position and the hyperemia to recede in the leg-down position. In debilitated patients, a rocking bed is a poor though possible substitute. I have found in early cases that local carbachol or methacholine (Mecholyl) iontophoresis over the dorsalis pedis artery has a salutary adjunctive effect, but to just what extent is difficult to judge. Coplanar shortwave diathermy and reflex heating over the lumbar sympathetics using a shortwave coil are also said to be helpful.

CONTRAST BATHS.   It may seem strange to list contrast baths under "exercise therapy" unless it is realized that they, in fact, produce gymnastics of the vascular tree. However, they should not be used in the presence of ischemia due to vascular disease. Indeed, in cases of arterial vascular deficiency, heat can precipitate gangrene. But in treating muscle pain when the muscle is deficient in blood supply from disuse, contrast baths are valuable and particularly suited for use in foot pain from this cause. I must stress again that contrast baths are contraindicated in arterial disease.

The time the foot is immersed in the hot water should be about twice the time spent in the cold water. The heat and cold should be tolerable to the normal hand. The duration of treatment should be 10 to 15 minutes.

Therapeutic Manipulation

Joint manipulation, being a method of moving joints passively, must be mentioned in this section if only to stress that the reestablishment of normal joint-play movements cannot be achieved in the presence of muscle activity. Therefore, it must not be considered as either a passive or an active exercise modality. However, functional exercises can be performed normally only when normal joint play is present.

RULES OF THERAPEUTIC MANIPULATION. Just as there are rules to be followed when examining a joint, so there are rules when manipulation is used to restore lost or impaired movements of joint play. For the most part the rules of technique for examination and for therapy are the same, just as the movements used in therapy are, for the most part, the same as those used in examination. These rules, now modified for therapy, are of sufficient importance to reiterate them as follows:

1. The patient must be relaxed, and each aspect of the joint being treated must be supported and protected from unguarded, painful movement that may otherwise occur in the course of the premanipulative positioning.
2. The therapist must be relaxed, and at no time must his grasp be painful to the patient; it must be firm and protective, not gripping and restrictive.
3. One joint should be mobilized at a time but in the foot, because of technical difficulties, it is not possible to achieve this perfection. In Chapter 4 in the topographical sections it is made clear when and why this rule has to be broken.

4. One movement at each joint is restored at a time.

5. In the performance of any one movement, one articular surface of the joint (or joints) being mobilized is moved upon that facet of the joint (or joints) being stablized. Thus there should always be one mobilizing force and one stabilizing force exerted during the performance of each therapeutic maneuver.

6. The extent of normal joint play can usually be assessed by examining the same joint in the opposite, unaffected foot, and the mobilizing force must never carry the joint being mobilized beyond this extent.

7. Forceful or abnormal movements must *never* be used. The movements of joint play must be carefully differentiated from those under control of the voluntary muscles. For instance, the medial tilt of the metatarsophalangeal joint of the big toe must not be confused with the voluntary movement of abduction, and the medial tilt of the subtalar joint, which is performed with the joint in long axis extension, must not be confused with inversion of the foot.

8. The manipulative movement used is a sharp springing thrust, push, or pull, and must be differentiated from a forceful movement, which denotes lack of control of it. An uncontrolled movement is an abnormal movement. If anesthesia is used to facilitate a therapeutic manipulation, the therapeutic movement should have no more force behind it while the patient is unconscious than would be used if he were conscious; in fact, usually it is unnecessary to use as much under these circumstances.

9. The springing movement is imparted to the joint only after taking up the slack in the joint to the point of pain. The movement is then taken through this pain point to the limit of normal movement. Thus, a mobilizing movement starts at, and goes through, the point at which pain is elicited and at which the examination technique was stopped.

10. In the presence of clinical signs of joint or bone inflammation or disease, no therapeutic movements should be undertaken.

USE OF ANESTHESIA IN MANIPULATION.   For some reason, controversy always arises when the subject of joint manipulation under anesthesia is mentioned. It is perfectly safe to manipulate a joint with a patient anesthetized providing no departure is made from the specific normal manipulative technique. Certainly it is dangerous to manipulate a joint with the aid of anesthesia if the manipulator applies more force to a joint than he would were the patient conscious, or if he moves the joint in an abnormal way or through any range of movement in the voluntary range of movement as described in the usual textbooks of anatomy. Anesthesia is used to obtain perfect control over a joint by eliminating resistant muscle spasm that cannot be eliminated by any other means. It is used to spare the patient pain. It is used to prevent the use of force, not to facilitate it.

LOCAL ANESTHESIA.   When a patient is unable to relax because of pain, local anesthetic solutions can be instilled into the joints of the foot and ankle and sufficiently reduce the pain so that a therapeutic manipulation can be performed. The use of local anesthetic solutions, however, has two drawbacks: (1) the patient should not move the joint through its voluntary range until sensation returns, which may take some hours; and (2) the patient not only experiences some psychological trauma when he hears the noise accompanying the manipulative movements but also has the feeling that the foot or the joint in the foot seems to be "dead." During recovery period from local anesthesia the mobilized joints tend to stiffen up again. Joint manipulation assisted by nerve blocks has the same associated problems.

INTRAARTICULAR INJECTION. Steroid preparations injected into the joints also produce a pain-free state to a greater or lesser degree, and during this period there is no reason why therapeutic manipulation should not be undertaken. I cannot see, however, that the use of steroids is of any especial benefit in joints in which there is joint dysfunction causing the symptoms of pain. The injection of any substance into a joint is, in my opinion, to be avoided unless it is necessary for some definite therapeutic object. The only cases of pyogenic pyarthrosis in adults that I have seen in practice have been caused by unnecessary introduction of needles into the joints.

I cannot feel that it is any more or less rational or safe to use general anesthesia to avoid pain during joint manipulation intended to restore normal movement and to achieve freedom from pain than it is to use it during the reduction of fractures and dislocations or, for that matter, to facilitate the extraction of a tooth.

9

Supports and Support Making

Most physicians now accept that shoes do not correct feet, but that feet correct shoes. Nevertheless, in every town and village it is possible to buy foot supports from either the local shoe repairman or the local store. Commercial foot supports, being mass produced to fit every foot, can hardly be expected to fit any. This is undoubtedly why such supports have their lumps and bumps made out of sponge rubber or other soft synthetic material. The support can then adapt fairly easily to the foot without causing additional pain.

There is only one condition in which a sponge-rubber device may be used with success, and that is infracalcaneal bursitis (page 127). In this condition treatment consists of raising and sloping the heel temporarily, and to achieve this there is a very satisfactory heel wedge* which can be put into any shoe. Providing the wedge does not slip forward in the shoe when it is put on, in which case the pain is increased, it helps to achieve relief in this condition.

To be effective, supports must fit not only the contours of the soles of the feet but also the contours of the innersoles of the shoes. Neither metal nor plastic nor wood-leather combinations can claim to provide both these necessary features, let alone be interchangeable from one pair of shoes to another. Even the best

* Manufactured by Scholl (Dr. Scholl's Foot Comfort Shoes).

supports made to fit one pair of shoes usually cannot be changed into another pair and still properly fit the contours of the feet and the different shoes.

Materials

I am sure that even most people trained to care for foot problems cannot really be satisfied with the usual materials used in fashioning supports. The public seems to expect supports, however, and they are provided with them, often, I think, at far too great expense. Fortunately, even the painful foot is sufficiently pliable to be able to adapt to most things that are placed in shoes.

However, a properly fashioned support positively relieves pain arising from many musculoskeletal causes. These supports are made either from cork (synthetic cork is more difficult to work) or from piano felt, which is a felt compressed by 50 pounds to the square inch. In shaping cork to fit, it is possible to whittle it by minute fractions of an inch, and it is also possible to bevel it down almost to paper thinness. This certainly cannot be done with metal or plastic; such accuracy can be approached using felt. Pressure caused by unresilient, poorly fitting supports produces muscle atrophy and sometimes nerve irritation which compound the pathological problem that they are prescribed to treat.

Principles of Successful Support Making

The first basic principle, from which success in support making follows, is arrived at by listening to the patient who has foot pain of a type in which a support might be expected to bring relief. This patient almost invariably states that his feet are comfortable at rest, and that pain develops only on standing or walking.

From this it should be easy to deduce that if a support is to ease foot pain, it must be so fashioned as to maintain the foot in the position of rest — or as near as possible to this position — when it is in function.

The second basic principle that is prerequisite to successful support making is to study the anatomical relationship of the metatarsal heads to each other. It is surprising how little attention is ever paid to this simple observation, or the metatarsal "pads" that are incorporated in most supports could not be shaped the way they are. Figure 9-1 demonstrates how anatomically inaccurate these pads are. The dotted line shows the shape of the usual metatarsal pad in relation to the metatarsal heads. The firm line shows the proper anatomical line that a support should follow. The instep lines also indicate the common error resulting from the insertion of a "cookie" under the instep, shown by a dotted line, as compared with the contour of the living instep indicated by the solid line. Footprints are misleading at best, as they are made with the foot in function — that is, in their painful state.

The usual concept of the division of the labor of weight bearing between the heads of the metatarsal bones is also misleading. I believe that pure weight bearing in function is divided equally between the head of the first metatarsal bone on the one hand, and the heads of the lateral four metatarsal bones equally on the other hand. Supporting this belief is the fact that the shafts of the four lateral metatarsal bones are virtually the same in diameter (allowing for their relatively decreasing lengths) and their heads are practically the same size. Compare these bones in the normal foot with the shape and sizes of the heads and shafts of the metatarsal bones in the atavistic foot — obviously an anatomically abnormal weight-bearing foot — in which the second metatarsal

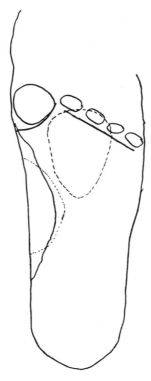

FIGURE 9-1.   The inaccuracies of commercial supports as they are usually made (*dotted lines*) when compared with the anatomical positions of the metatarsal heads (*solid line*). Compare also the usual "cookie" to support the "longitudinal arch" (*dotted line*) when compared with the true elevation of the instep (*solid line*).

has to do more than its share of weight bearing; clearly, its shaft is broader and its head larger to cope with these added stresses. In assessing these observations, the reader should understand that I do not disagree with the usually accepted view of how weight bearing in ambulation is placed on the metatarsal heads as the body weight comes forward over the advanced foot in a serial manner from the outer to the inner side.

Design or Blueprint

In assessing a foot for which a support is to be made, it is necessary to observe it at rest, and this is best done with the patient in the supine recumbent position. The foot from the back of the calcaneus to the front of the tarsal bones is flat. From this point the forefoot drops forward. The degree of the forefoot drop depends on the resiliency and relative length of the Achilles tendon, on the resiliency and length of the plantar fascia and of the long and short plantar ligaments, and, to a lesser extent, on the resiliency of the intrinsic muscles of the foot and on the resiliency and length of the long tendons of the extrinsic muscles of the foot. The weight-bearing aspects of the metatarsal heads are noted at the ball of the foot, and a measure of whether these are their normal weight-bearing aspects is assessed by whether or not the toes are dorsiflexed in this position of rest. If they are dorsiflexed, it is almost certain that those parts of the metatarsal heads which are exposed to weight bearing are not the parts designed for this purpose.

One must also realize that the positions of the metatarsal heads in the long axis and in the width of the foot, together with their anatomical relationships, are going to change as soon as the patient stands up. The metatarsal heads are then no longer in their position of painlessness. Yet it is necessary to mark their rest position in fashioning a support; it is also necessary to aim at filling up the space between the contours of the foot at rest and the unchangeable contours of the inside of the shoe.

From these observations it should be obvious that any forces that alter the rest contours of the foot while a pattern is being made are bound to change the anatomy of the foot from its painless rest position. This vitiates the methods of taking impressions of the foot, whether this is done by pouring a positive sculpture from a plaster cast or by shaping the support from the negative mold of the standing impression of the foot in plaster. In the former case, the person making the cast is holding the foot in the position which *he thinks* is the correct position of the foot; in the latter case, the foot is outlined in its painful functional position. In parenthesis, it should be noted here that adequate supports cannot be made in pairs (as most commercial supports are sold), as invariably no two feet of any individual are the same in length, breadth, or contour.

The bespoke shoemaker is the artist at designing supports. He builds from blueprints just as an architect does. Instructions for drafting accurate patterns from which proper supports can be made out of cork or felt are to be found in Chapter 11. However, in making shoes there is no need to shape the undersurface of the platform as must be done when building a support to fit into a preexisting shoe. Because of this difference and because proper fashioning is so important, the cardinal techniques are described here, with the added needs required in support making, in contrast to shoe making.

Platform Support

The Pattern. CONTOUR OF INNER ASPECT OF THE FOOT. The elevation of the contour of the inner aspect of the foot is drawn from two positions. The first is with the patient supine and recumbent. A duraluminum strip is molded to the inner aspect of the foot at rest from behind the heel to beyond the head of the first metatarsal head distally (Fig. 9-2). The contour of the metal strip is then traced onto the paper on which the rest of the pattern is to be drawn.

HEIGHT OF HEEL.   As the optimum benefit of a support partially depends on the height of the shoe heel needed for the best weight-bearing distribution in the patient's foot, this is now measured from the upright duraluminum strip. The heel part of the foot must be maintained parallel to the ground, so the heel of the metal contour is raised from the ground until it is horizontal and the distance of the metal from the ground is measured (Fig. 9-3); this is the optimum heel height for that foot. On a

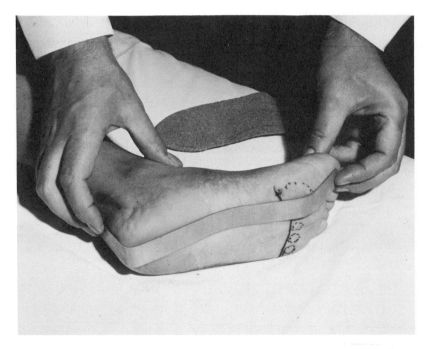

FIGURE 9-2.   Making an elevation pattern of the contour of the inner border of the foot (the instep) using a duraluminum strip. Figure 9-3 illustrates how this is then used to determine the optimum heel height of a shoe for this foot.

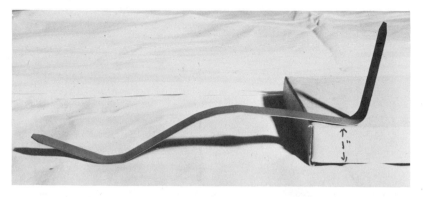

FIGURE 9-3. The duraluminum strip removed from the foot. The heel impression is raised until the posterior contour is parallel with the ground. The height of the heel part from the ground is a measure of the optimal shoe heel height.

store-bought shoe, it should be remembered that no lift more than ½ inch high can be added to it without causing a breakdown of the shoe, so anything higher than a 1-inch heel requirement must be added by using a platform support inside the shoe; in practice this cannot be more than ¼ inch high, and even then a cuff may have to be added to the quarter of the shoe so that it still accommodates the heel of the foot.

POSITION OF METATARSAL HEADS AT REST. The skin on the sole of the foot is now marked with wet ink in three places: (1) just behind the head of the first metatarsal bone; (2) just behind the head of the second metatarsal bone; and (3) just behind the head of the fifth metatarsal bone. Then, using the flat of a nib dipped in ink, the marks at the backs of the fifth and second metatarsal bones are joined by a straight line. This line indicates the position of the lateral four metatarsal heads. Then the marks behind the second and the first metatarsal heads are joined by a line curving around the head of the first metatarsal bone (Fig. 9-4). While these lines are still wet, the patient

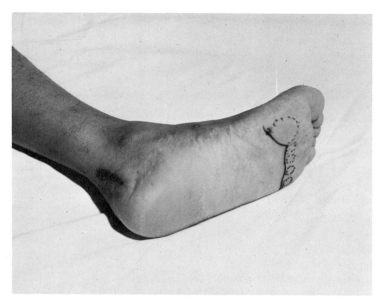

FIGURE 9-4.   The foot (photographically foreshortened) showing
the positions of the metatarsal heads at rest and the wet ink lines on
which the flat pattern is based drawn on the skin. Though the bones
move when the patient stands, the ink line remains where the metatarsal heads were at rest.

stands down on the pattern paper with his weight on his heel. He
then carefully transfers his weight forward onto the forefoot,
without raising his heel from the ground, and remains standing
in this position while the foot outline is drawn. In outlining the
foot, the designer must take great care to hold the pencil upright
at all times. The sole of the foot bevels in all around before making contact with the paper, and if the pencil is slanted in or out,
the platform pattern will end up either too narrow or too wide.

INSTEP ELEVATION.   While still standing thus, the second outline of the elevation of the inner aspect of the foot is made. The
pencil point is placed just proximal to the head of the first meta-

tarsal bone and is swept around under the sole of the foot on its medial side backward until it emerges again at the front of the heel. This outlines the instep elevation and indicates that part of the sole which does not come into contact with the paper, thereby giving the designer the flat elevation pattern. Then the patient raises the foot straight up, leaving the design on the paper as illustrated in Figure 9-5.

Fashioning the Support.   The paper pattern is placed on a slab of cork ½ inch thick with a piece of carbon paper between it and

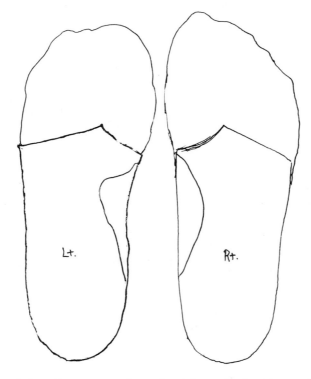

FIGURE 9-5.   The pattern of a pair of feet, obtained by tracing in the manner described in the text. The method of determining the lines for the rest positions of the metatarsal heads is shown in Figure 9-4.

the cork. The outlines of the pattern are then traced through the carbon paper onto the cork and the cork pattern is cut out.

SHAPING THE CORK-FOOT SURFACE. *For the Lateral Four Metatarsal Heads.* In Figure 9-6 the cork pattern is shown somewhat foreshortened, with those parts of the cork which have to be filed away outlined. A cobbler's rasp (Fig. 9-7, 9-11) is used for this; its filing edges are coarse and fine, and one end is rounded and the other flat. On the other side the filing surfaces are reversed: under the coarse, rounded end is the fine, flat end; under the fine, flat end is the coarse, rounded end.

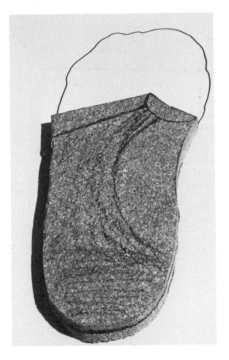

FIGURE 9-6. The cut-out support from the cork slab, showing its upper surface. Distally lines are drawn indicating those areas to be rasped away to support the metatarsal heads. Proximal to these lines, the shaded area has to be rasped away in a gentle slope laterally, but the heel area must remain flat. The instep support remains unshaded and is left alone. The cobbler's rasp is illustrated in Figures 9-7 and 9-11.

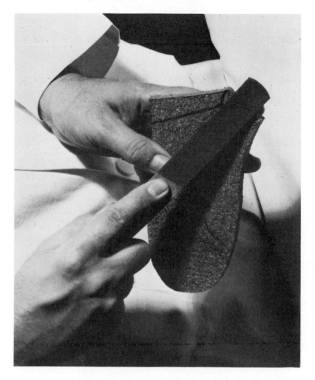

FIGURE 9-7.   The coarse, curved surface of the cobbler's rasp being used to fashion the cradle for the head of the first metatarsal
bone.

The front shelf on which the heads of the four lateral metatarsal bones will rest is filed away at an angle of about 45 degrees widening somewhat from its medial to its lateral aspect. The
coarse, flat aspect of the rasp is used to do this. The shelf is filed
down to nothing at its leading edge, the anterior-inferior border.

For the First Metatarsal Head.   The cradle for the head of
the first metatarsal bone is filed away using the coarse, curved end
of the rasp, which is swiveled around as the cradle takes shape.
Figure 9-7 illustrates the use of the rasp during this phase.

For the Platform and Heel.   This part of the fashioning of the
support is the most difficult to describe, as it requires freehand
shaping. The coarse, flat end of the rasp is used. The shaded

areas (see Fig. 9-6) have to be filed down, sloping away laterally from the firm line drawn from the contour of the instep. But while the anterolateral part must slope downward and outward, the heel part posteriorly must remain flat and horizontal.

The finished shaping of the foot side of the support is shown in Figure 9-8. Note that the corners should be rounded off. The peak between the cradle for the big toe and the shelf for the other toes has been made smooth. The proximal upper edges of the respective shelves have been rounded off. All this finishing work is done with the fine-filing aspects of the rasp.

SHAPING THE CORK-SHOE SURFACE. The undersurface of the cork must be curved to fit the long axis arch of the sole of the

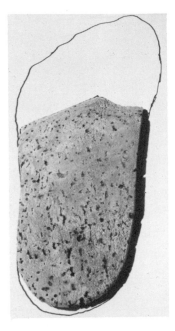

FIGURE 9-8. The foot aspect of the cork platform support in its finished state before fitting. Compare with Figure 9-6 (before support is fashioned), and note how the corners and edges have been rounded off.

shoe, but that part of the cork supporting the metatarsal heads must be higher than the platform itself to fit the "drop-away" of the front of the shoe. This lifts the metatarsal heads and holds up the natural drop of the forefoot. Figure 9-9 shows the under-surface of the cork, which is lined to show the areas of cork to be filed away (the picture again is somewhat foreshortened). From the horizontal line across the front of the cork, nearly half a thickness of the cork is cut away backward to the heel to the depth of the line drawn around the sides and heel of the cork. The remaining surface must be flat and horizontal. From the

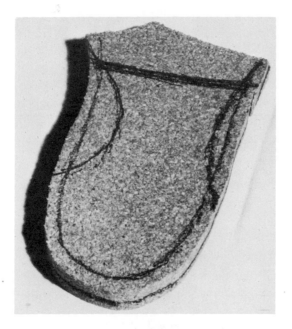

FIGURE 9-9. The undersurface of the platform support in the rough. The drop-away of the forefoot is maintained by the cork distal to the heavy horizontal line, which remains untouched. The line all around the cork indicates where the beveling must be done. The line around the edge of the cork shows the depth to which the platform must be filed away. The curved medial line indicates the cork that must be filed away medially to fit the waist of the shoe. The curved lateral line indicates how the lateral part of the waist of the cork must be shaped.

front line the cut-away follows a gentle curve extending backward for about an inch, and is smoothed using the curved end of
the rasp. Two curved lines, one on the medial side and one on
the lateral side, will be noted. Using the coarse, curved end of the
rasp, cradles are now filed away to paper thinness at the upper
aspect of the support, sloping gently toward the middle of the
cork. The cradles so formed accommodate the instep arches of
the waist at the junction of the shoe's insole and upper. The
whole bottom of the cork is then smoothed with the flat, fine
end of the rasp. Finally, the edge of the cork is beveled in all
around from the upper outer edges to make it adapt to the welt-
ing-in of the upper of the quarter and vamp into the foundation
of the shoe.

FITTING THE CORK TO THE SHOE.   The cork is then placed in
the shoe and should fit flat on the sole without rocking or sloping
from one side to the other. If rocking occurs, the under side of
the cork must be whittled away until the cork fits without rocking. If there is a side-to-side slope, this has to be corrected to
avoid foot inversion or eversion.

FITTING THE CORK TO THE FOOT.   The support is now fitted
to the sole of the foot, as shown in Figure 9-10. In doing this, it
must be noted that the back of the heel of the cork is in line with
the posterior limit of the calcaneus where the Achilles tendon inserts, not forward to the place where the undersurface of the
foot first come in contact with the cork. The patient stands on the
cork and notes any ridges, bumps, or knife-like edges. These are
filed away. It cannot be stressed too strongly that a single sweep
of the rasp may be sufficient to correct a bump that feels like
a mountain to the patient. If too much is filed away, it can never
be put back.

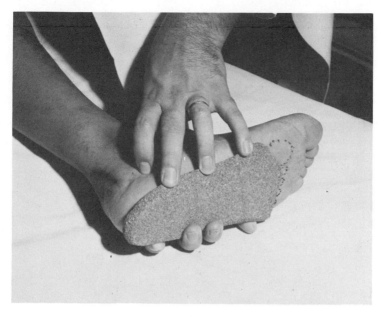

FIGURE 9-10. The finished cork platform support being fitted to the foot. The illustration shows the shoe side of the cork, which is fashioned as described in Figure 9-9; its finished appearance is well shown. Note that the back of the cork extends beyond the back of the sole of the foot so that a plumb line dropped from the most posterior part of the calcaneus is above it. This is to ensure the cork fitting the back of the shoe correctly.

FITTING THE SHOE AND SUPPORT TO THE FOOT. The shoe, with the support in it, is put on the patient's stockinged foot. The fitter uses his thumb to hold the support back in the heel of the shoe. (The thumb fits very easily in the medial aspect of the waist of the shoe even with the foot in it, providing the laces are loose.) The heel must be eased into the shoe with a shoehorn. Then the laces are tied, and the patient stands. Lumps, bumps, and knife-like edges may again be felt, and again these must be whittled away — but only a very little at a time. When standing is comfortable, the patient walks, and other adjustments may have to be made. When all is comfortable, the support is glued into the

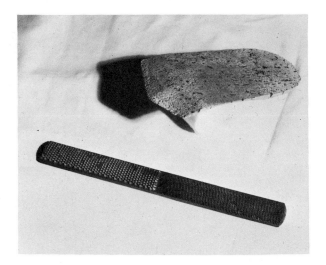

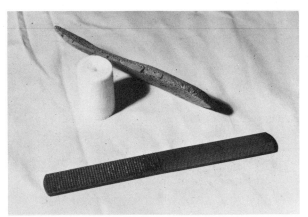

FIGURE 9-11.   Two views of the finished support.

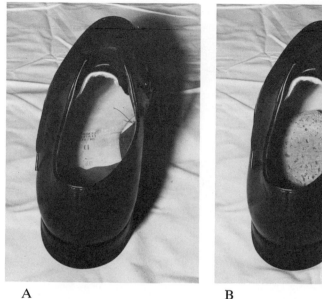
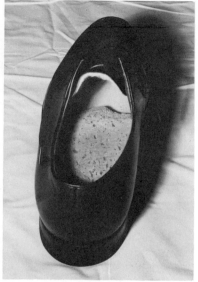

A   B

FIGURE 9-12.   The shoe without the support (A) and with the
support in place (B).

shoe and covered by a leather lining. To accommodate the thickness of the leather lining, a fraction of the cork is filed away from
the bottom of the whole cork. Figure 9-11 shows the finished
support, and Figure 9-12 shows the shoe without the support and
with it in place.

THE SHOE IN WHICH THE SUPPORT IS PLACED.   The store-
bought shoe which is to be adapted to a painful foot by the use of
a platform support always has to be 1 or 1½ sizes larger than
the shoe usually worn by the patient, if he was wearing a large
enough shoe in the first place. It must also be a size wider. A
quarter heel cuff may have to be added to keep the heel of the
foot in the shoe, and a tongue pad may have to be inserted to

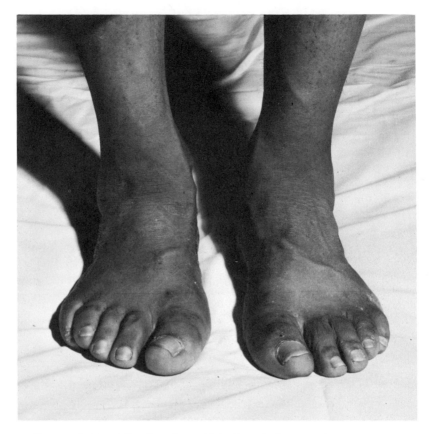

FIGURE 9-13.   The feet for which the platform cork support was made. The support was needed for the left foot; the right foot was free of pain. The discrepencies between the two feet are well illustrated in Figure 9-5.

keep the heel back in the shoe. The heel height has yet to be adjusted.

With the platform in the shoe there is already a new heel height, which is the height of the external heel added to the height of the cork at the heel. If more is needed, a leather wedge is added to the external heel, always remembering that no wedge measuring more than ½ inch posteriorly and sloping to ¼ inch anteriorly can be tolerated externally by the shoe. The shoe heel may need lowering.

The cork platform support in these illustrations was made for the left foot of the pair of feet illustrated in Figure 9-13. The right foot was pain free. The discrepencies between the two feet are well illustrated in Figure 9-5, yet only the one foot was painful. The heel height of the unaltered shoe may have to be changed to prevent gait abnormalities from developing, but this is not always necessary.

Anterior Metatarsal-Head Support

The anterior metatarsal-head support is fashioned in exactly the same manner as the platform support and can be made out of cork or piano felt. The difference is that the platform part of the support is cut away from immediately behind the heavy transverse line that is shown in the illustration for shaping the cork to the shoe (Fig. 9-9), and the part that goes backward into the middle of the foot is cut in a rounded-off triangular shape and filed away from the undersurface, sloping from the full thickness in front to a paper-thin edge proximally.

FITTING THE SUPPORT TO THE FOOT. The support is placed under and just proximal to the metatarsal heads, as in fitting the

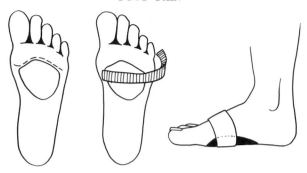

FIGURE 9-14.   The anterior metatarsal-head support (*left*), and how
it is fitted to the foot before being incorporated into the shoe (*center
and right*).

platform support (Fig. 9-14). It can be taped to the foot using
adhesive tape, and the patient stands on it. Any lumps or bumps
are noted and these are whittled away. (If felt is used, this requires a razor-sharp cobbler's knife — in fact, the whole of a felt
support has to be fashioned using one of these knives.) The support is then carefully placed back on the foot — it rotates out of
place very easily — and, if it is comfortable, the foot with the
support on it is very carefully put into the shoe whose laces are
absolutely loose so that the upper can be opened as wide as possible. The heel is eased into the shoe with the use of a shoehorn.
The adhesive attachment of the support to the foot is so unstable
that this can be done only once with each taping. Again, any
lumps and bumps are removed.

When comfortable, the support is ready to be incorporated
into the shoe, and this is the most critical procedure. The support
is again carefully put on the foot. A thin cork insole is now
placed under the entire sole of the foot beneath the support. It
does not matter where the front of this cork insole is, as long as its
heel is far enough back on the heel of the foot so that its edge is
proximal to the foot heel, so that it is under the place where a
plumb line dropped from the Achilles tubercle of the calcaneus

posteriorly would hit the ground. This means that the insole heel edge will be up against the back of the heel of the shoe. If this is not the case, when finished the support is always too proximal. The support, held firmly against the sock insole, is now removed and outlined in ink on the insole. But the support, of course, is on the wrong side of the sock insole, the front of which is now cut off, carefully following the drawn outline of the leading edge of the support. Then the support is transferred to the undersurface of the sock insole and glued onto it. The utmost care must be taken to ensure that the leading edge of the support is exactly contiguous with the leading edge of the sock insole.

For final fitting, the support can be handled exactly like a full platform support. It is placed in the shoe and held back in the heel by the fitter's thumb inserted into the upper on the medial aspect of the waist while the foot is eased into the shoe, using a shoehorn. Minor alterations can still be made by whittling on the exposed undersurface of the cork or felt. When it is perfectly comfortable, it is glued to the insole of the shoe and covered with a thin leather liner which is glued over it from heel to toe. The heel height of the shoe may have to be adjusted upward or downward to produce the optimal benefit to the painful foot.

10

Shoes—General Considerations

Throughout this book a deliberate attempt has been made to avoid the term *arch* because of the strong tendency of those who deal with foot problems to blame so much of foot pain on problems of the arches. True, it makes it easy when talking to the layman about his feet. He thinks he understands what is being discussed because we are forever being exposed to the term by shoe salesmen, in advertisements by shoe manufacturers in newspapers, magazines, radio, and television, and by salesmen of supports, shoe repairmen, podiatrists, family doctors, and orthopedic surgeons. Arches fall, feet are flat, arch supports are made.

In talking of the feet and shoes, however, I have to fall back on the use of the word *arch* for descriptive purposes and for word economy. But it must not be thought that its use in any way implies a reversal of my thesis that consideration of the longitudinal arches and anterior metatarsal arch per se is any substitute for determining the pathological causes of foot pain in patients. Far from it. "Correction" of arches more often causes symptoms than relieves them, and corrective shoes seldom, if ever, correct anything in the foot; the foot invariably corrects the shoe, which is a pain-producing process in itself.

Correct Design of Shoes

LENGTH.   A shoe size is ⅓ inch measured on a shoe stick; shoe stores use other expensive sorts of apparatus. But the measurement is not taken from heel to toe in thirds of inches; the shoe sizes start to be measured from an arbitrarily advanced point on the shoe stick (3⅓ inches in the United States and 4⅓ inches in England) in front of the heel. The arbitrary point to change from children to adult sizes is when the foot reaches child's size 13.

BREADTH.   The reference to shoe widths as A through E is an artificial, though maybe convenient, designation referring to the width across the ball of the foot. This is better measured in inches and compared to the width of the foot while weight bearing. The proper width of a shoe is ¼ inch less than the width of the foot, measured while weight bearing across the heads of the metatarsals; this ¼ inch should not be taken off from one side or the other but should be subtracted as ⅛ inch from each side.

THE HEEL.   The proper height of a shoe heel is that which keeps the hind part of the heel of the foot horizontal with the ground in standing. The way to measure the heel height of a shoe which is correct for a foot is explained on page 200. The heel must form a broad base for weight bearing. The set of the heel is important. Any tendency for the angle of the heel at the forepart on the inner side to turn inward means that the wearer tends to evert the foot with each step — a pain-producing situation. Any heel less wide than the waist part of the sole of the shoe makes balance precarious and causes constant strain on the supporting structures of the ankle (and indeed the knee, hip, and low back) and may be responsible for pain. Anything approaching a spike heel has to be accompanied by pain in the human heel resting on the spike, in any of the joints of the leg, and in the low back or other part of the spine; indeed, the wearing of a spike heel may even be a cause of headaches, or at least pain referred from the neck into the head which is described by a patient as headaches. The correct heel height is proportional to the length and resiliency of the Achilles tendon.

THE SOLE.   The shoe sole must be flat and should slope only gently upward distal to the metatarsal heads. A sole with a marked upward slope distally causes a constant dorsiflexion strain of the metatarsophalangeal joints and promotes a "digging in" stress of the metatarsal heads into the sole, with resulting pain. Any convexity of the sole from side to side results in a tendency to pinch the metatarsal heads together, a common cause of meta-tarsalgia (see page 111).

THE UPPER.   The correct adjustments of the last over which the upper is stretched is vital to the proper fit of the shoe. The fit of the shoe eventually is determined by the last and not the shape of the upper — the leather fitted over it. The inner side must be straight from the "waist" of the shoe to the tip of the big toe. Distal to this it may safely be shaped "to taste." It must not slope outward and downward across the dorsal aspect of the metatarsophalangeal joints, or it compresses the lateral four joints. There must be room beneath the upper for each individual toe to rest flat in long axis extension and in a straight line with the axis of each metatarsal bone. The upper should be snug, however, just behind the heads of the first and fifth metatarsals. There must be space for complete freedom of movement and expansion distal to this. Toe stiffeners to support the uppers are needed but toe caps are overlays, cosmetic, and frequently a cause of pain over the dorsum of the toes. Lacing of the upper is essential to shoe comfort. The Bal (Balmoral) shoe is laced across "V" tabs with an underlying free "tongue." Blucher (Derby) shoes are laced across the free wing tabs with a cover tongue. Bal shoes require more stitching, and though smarter, more causes of pain are likely to arise from a vamp of this design than from the vamp of a Blucher shoe. The ultimate comfort of the shoe still depends on its being long enough.

THE QUARTER. The quarter refers to the hind part of the shoe, which must grasp the heel firmly to prevent it from sliding up and down in the shoe with walking. A heel stiffener is used partially for this and partially to prevent breakdown of the leather. In store shoes, however, if the vamp is broad enough, the quarter is seldom narrow enough; this heel problem can be overcome, however, by incorporating a tongue pad which helps to keep the heel of the foot back snugly in the heel of the shoe. Heavy stitching at the back of the quarter, unless well protected, may irritate the Achilles tendon structures. The insole of the quarter must be gently concave; however, too deep a concavity of the inside at the heel is conducive to the production of calcaneal bursitis. The waists are arched and the heels slightly concave.

THE SHANK. The steel shank, such a vaunted feature of "orthopedic shoes," simply serves to prevent breakdown of the sole of the shoe, thereby ensuring a longer life of the shoe. Cheap shoes have cardboard or maybe wood-plastic shanks, and the shoe waist is rapidly destroyed; the shoe upper creases and cracks early, and the shoe is worn out prematurely. Of course, a properly placed steel shank maintains the longitudinally arched shape of the shoe, adding to its supportive features but not to its "corrective" features. A shoe with a steel shank is obviously a better, longer lasting shoe than one without it. Its incorporation is of economic rather than therapeutic benefit.

THE LINING.   The lining of the shoe must be of good quality leather smoothly applied to the sole, vamp, and quarter. Creases in the lining are frequent causes of foot pain.

Materials

Calf leather remains the best material from which shoes are fashioned. It is pliable, yet when shaped, it maintains its shape and supportive functions well. Kid leather, which has the advantage of being lighter, stretches readily and loses its design and its supportive functions. Pigskin has recently come into vogue in shoe making. However, it stiffens and cracks after wetting. If pigskins were cured by using glutenaldehyde, this problem might be overcome. A rubber heel covering the leather heel absorbs some of the shock of impact when the shoe strikes the ground in walking and spares the human heel within the shoe. It also has the advantage of being cheaply replaced when it is worn down. Plastic is not as resilient as calf leather, nor can it be molded as accurately in lasting. It does not breathe as well as leather, so heat and sweating of the foot may become a problem.

Socks and Stockings

Hose which are too tight cause as much foot trouble as too tight shoes. Cheap hose with rough seams provoke as much trouble as heavy shoe stitching protected only by cheap shoe lining. Too large hose may wrinkle and produce pain problems just as wrinkled cheap shoe lining does.

Irregularity of Feet

Few people have two feet of the same size and shape. So, when choosing a pair of shoes, it is wise to select a pair large enough for the bigger foot. The shoe worn on the smaller foot can be readily adjusted by wearing an insole in it (or a thicker sock) and by the addition of a tongue pad if necessary to keep the heel of the foot back in the heel of the shoe. With gross foot irregularity, many shoe stores will provide mismatched shoes.

Shoe Adjustments

Except for wearing an insole and a tongue pad to hold the foot heel back in the shoe heel, as mentioned in the foregoing paragraph, attempts to block up bottoms of the soles and fill in arch cavities between the shoe and foot can be successful only on a hit-or-miss basis. Calf uppers can be stretched with a degree of success, but not to any great extent, to accommodate a hump or a bump. If a store-bought shoe is to be used to accommodate any form of added support, it must be wider and longer than that usually worn. To accommodate a full platform support, the shoe usually has to be 1½ sizes longer and 1 size wider. To heighten it, a cuff may have to be added to the back of the quarter to keep the heel of the foot in the shoe.

Heel Adaptations. RAISING THE HEEL.   The heel of a store-bought shoe can be raised to compensate for Achilles tendon insufficiency, but not more than by a wedge that, in the longitudinal plane, measures ½ inch posteriorly and slopes forward to ¼ inch anteriorly. This provides a maximum central heel lift of about ⅜ inch. The average height of a man's shoe heel is ½ inch when the shoe is bought. The wedging is important. A "square" lift catches on walking and raises the sole of the shoe from the ground, and this produces early breakdown of the sole. Furthermore, a higher adjustment produces too great an incline from heel to toe and causes the foot to slide forward in the shoe; this creates pain in the forefoot by altering weight bearing on the metatarsal heads and in the toes from their impingement on the toe of the shoe. If a higher heel than this is required, a platform support within the shoe must also be used to keep the heel part of the foot horizontal and to redistribute the weight bearing of the metatarsal heads. If the heel of one shoe is raised, it is usually proper to raise the heel of the other shoe even with a physiological (not pathological) inequality of leg length. Patients have adapted to most "physiological" postural defects, and if unilateral adjustments are made, they develop symptoms because they have to make a new adaptation in structures less resilient because of normal aging processes.

WEDGING THE HEEL.   Raising of the medial side of the heel of a shoe by wedging, usually by not more than ⅛ inch, is commonly prescribed as a panacea for foot and ankle problems. Like using sponge rubber or elastic bandages for supports, empirical prescription treats the psyche of the patient rather than the pathological condition giving rise to his symptoms. However, medial heel wedging may help correction of ankle pronation and assist in the relief of foot pain secondary to this if, and only if, all the

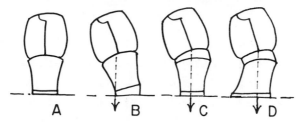

FIGURE 10-1. The correct and incorrect methods of applying wedging to the heel of a shoe. A. The normal shoe. B. Addition of a wedge to the bottom of the heel, which throws off the whole shoe. C. The wedge better placed between the heel and the sole. D. The correct placement of the wedge between the sole and the heel, with the heel flat medially to compensate for the instability of the shoe which results from weight bearing over an uncompensated wedge. (From J. B. Mennell, *Physical Treatment by Mobilization and Massage* [5th ed.]. London: Churchill, 1945.)

other reeducative measures advocated in Chapter 7 are prescribed as well. When medial wedges are prescribed, the shoemaker must add them in such a way that, when in place, the lower end of the posterior seam of the quarter is vertically above the heel (Fig. 10-1) when the adapted heel is flat on the ground. Also, the outside side of the heel should be curved to broaden the base of the heel and counteract instability that the wedge might otherwise cause. The extent of the curve is indicated in Figure 10-1D. Its outer edge should extend to rest below the top of the upper or even beyond. Medial heel wedges of this kind can be used with advantage as an adjunct to all the other modalities described in the severely strained, so-called painful flatfoot syndrome, but it cannot be of help with an anatomical flatfoot which, as has been remarked earlier, is most frequently painless.

THE THOMAS HEEL. This classic heel modification has the advantage of increasing the weight-bearing surface of the heel and was originally designed theoretically to support the talonavicular joint which was thought to be the key problem of the foot with "fallen arches." Though frequently used, especially in children's shoes, it is of doubtful therapeutic value. A Thomas heel may help a patient with foot eversion. A reverse Thomas heel may help a patient with foot inversion. Figure 10-4 on page 227 shows a modified Thomas heel.

Sole Adaptations. THE METATARSAL BAR.   A metatarsal bar is in reality a first-aid device used to relieve the metatarsophalangeal joints of function by allowing the shoe to rock over the bar instead of requiring the phalanges to dorsiflex. Thus it has a use in the treatment of fractures of the phalanges and metatarsals, especially when ambulation is first resumed. Its proper placement, with its forward edge behind the metatarsal heads, its proper angulation across the sole of the shoe, also related to the metatarsal heads, and the proper clearance which it provides — that is, ⅛ inch (Fig. 10-2) — are all essential to its effectiveness. Metatarsal bars wear down very quickly and are of benefit only for short periods. In the long-term treatment of metatarsalgia arising from metatarsal joint problems, they have little use.

THE ROCKER BOTTOM.   This sole adaptation, when used together with a properly fashioned platform support, is invaluable in the relief of pain from hallux rigidus or following surgical procedures that have included metatarsophalangeal joint fusion for any reason. The shoe can now take up any lost function of dorsiflexion of these joints in ambulation. The peak of the rocker is proximal to the metatarsophalangeal joints (Fig. 10-3).

Hauser Shoe Adaptations.   I have been impressed with the Hauser shoe modifications used in the treatment of valgus of the subtalar joint and of the pain associated with it. Pain from this condition may loosely be attributed to the flatfoot resulting

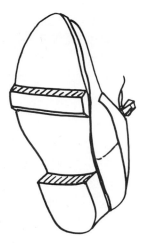

FIGURE 10-2. The metatarsal bar. Its proper placement behind the heads of the metatarsal bones is essential for success in its use. See Figure 10-3 to compare its effectiveness with that of the well-constructed rocker bottom.

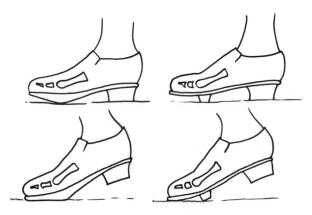

FIGURE 10-3. On the left, the effective use of a rocker bottom, sparing the metatarsophalangeal joints in walking. The two pictures on the right show, in an exaggerated way, the less efficient metatarsal bar. (From J. B. Mennell, *Physical Treatment by Mobilization and Massage* [5th ed.]. London: Churchill, 1945.)

from the mechanical disadvantage in the joint. The foot has to be maintained in a "rolled-over" position medially. The flatfootedness is apparent, not real, and it is therefore correctable. But while it persists there is marked ligament and tendon strain from which the pain surely arises. Thus, part of the treatment must be directed at these structures too. The methods of physical therapy to be used have been already outlined.

The Hauser shoe corrections can be made only on shoes from which the metal shank has been removed. Thus, the prerequisite of other shoe modification is here excepted. The inner side of the heel of the shankless shoe is raised by ¼ inch, to throw the heel from valgus into varus. The shape of the heel is a near–Thomas heel. Then to ensure that the inner side of the anterior part of the foot shall be lower than the outer side, a transverse but curved bar is added to the sole of the shoe. The bar is constructed so that it forms an inclined plane which is higher on the outer side than on the medial side. The bar ends behind the head of the fourth metatarsal bone. The anterior curve of the bar must be behind the metatarsal heads. Figure 10-4 illustrates the placing of and the mechanism of the modifications. In reality these modifications on the outside of the shoe simulate the platform support described in Chapter 9 on the inside of the shoe. They are more simple and are adequate for the average patient, perhaps, but less lasting and adequate for the problem patient.

The Hauser modified shoe is not effective unless the patient is taught to walk properly in them. Normal gait then becomes a corrective exercise. The flatfoot gait — that is, with both feet turned out and with the feet shifting rather than giving propulsion, and with exaggerated lumbar lordosis instead of a rolled-under pelvis (Chapter 3) — is usual in such a patient and must be overcome. The patient must be taught to roll his pelvis under him, to pull himself up as tall as possible, and to turn the toes in

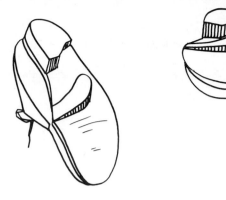

FIGURE 10-4. The Hauser shoe and adaptations. Note that the metal shank must be removed for these alterations to work. The heel is a modified Thomas heel. (From E. D. W. Hauser, *Surg. Clin. N. Amer.* 25:136–160, 1945.)

so that the feet point straight ahead. He must be taught to place the heel on the ground with the foot in dorsiflexion at heel strike. Holding this dorsiflexion, the body weight rolls over the heel, keeping the knee extended. Then as the body weight transfers forward, it is gradually transmitted to the outer side of the foot until the forward bar rolls it back onto the head of the first metatarsal and push-off occurs normally. Walking in shoes with Hauser modifications must be practiced initially for short periods or strain and pain from the corrected use of the foot will ensue, and the patient will revert readily to the bad old habits in an attempt to relieve them. Once a patient becomes accustomed to the new function of his feet, he is addicted to the Hauser shoe.

11

Shoe Making—Special Shoes

Because of the virtual disappearance of the bespoke shoemaker, we accept as footwear for the relief of painful or deformed feet (or both) such things as "molded shoes," "space shoes," and, more happily, shoes with the Ripple Sole.

Ripple Sole

The Ripple Sole was invented in 1949 during research at the University of Southern California aimed at developing an improved paratrooper boot, and credit is given for it to Nathan Hack, a retired shoemaker, working with Lawrence E. Morehouse, Ph.D., who had charge of the project. With the Ripple Sole, the kinetic energy of the mass of the foot and shoe is taken up by the first wave of the ripple. The sole then distorts, absorbing the energy, so that the wearer does not suffer a sharp, unyielding blow at each heel strike. As the weight is then transferred from heel to toe, each successive forward ripple picks up the load and distorts in the same manner. By suitable measuring devices, it has been shown that the "ripple principle" cuts down the peak shock of ground contact by as much as 40 percent. When one realizes that the peak downward force at heel strike may be as much as 120 percent of the body weight, a 160-pound man averaging 19,500 steps a day receives 3,705,000 pounds of pressure in repeated jolts. The shock-absorber qualities of the Ripple Sole cannot help but be of enormous benefit to the patient with foot pain. However, if the upper of the shoe still does not fit the foot, and if the insole still does not fit the contours and weight-bearing points of the foot, this tackles only a fraction of the patient's problem. It is certainly better than nothing, however. Other advantages of the Ripple Sole are in prolonged standing, when it assists the dynamic principles of posture, its nonskid properties, foot insulation without loss of ventilation, and protection of the foot from crushing in industrial accidents, for instance.

Space Shoes and Molded Shoes

The comfort of these shoes is probably due to the fact that they are made so roomy and have resilient insoles and outsoles that may incorporate to a degree some of the good features of the Ripple Sole, together with the well-known fact, first realized in World War I, that the infantryman is most comfortable in the least-shaped infantry boot. With the lack of availability of the bespoke shoe, I suppose this is the best we have to offer patients if we are not prepared to fashion supports ourselves, fit them properly into store-bought shoes, and institute proper therapy programs for foot rehabilitation.

Bespoke Shoes

There is no substitute ideally, when dealing with severe pain problems in the foot, for the bespoke hand-made shoe. These shoes are the creation of artists. Just as a painter can paint only an average portrait from a photograph but a living one from life, for a shoemaker to create his best shoe, he must see the living feet that his shoes have to fit. However, he can fit an averagely difficult foot from adequate patterns.

It is almost useless to expect a "special" shoe to be made from either a plaster cast or a plaster mold. In the case of the plaster cast someone is "molding" the foot in the cast and holding it in a position that *he thinks* is normal; this can only lead to fundamental error. Less well can a shoe for pain relief be built from a plaster cast. The impression of the foot in the mold is the position and shape of the foot in its pain-producing shape — that of weight bearing. The foundation of effective pain-relieving shoes must be a profile of the foot in its *pain-free* state — that is, at rest. The true artist works from a paper pattern as an architect does.

The Pattern. POSITION OF THE METATARSAL HEADS AT REST. The first thing essential to building a shoe is to know the position of the metatarsal heads at rest. As they move forward and apart with weight bearing, some way of noting this must be devised. This is easily achieved by marking their position at rest on the skin of the sole of the foot. It is not necessary to outline bones. To record the rest position of the metatarsal heads, the head of the first metatarsal bone is palpated and a mark is made on the skin immediately proximal to it — that is, just behind the head. Then the head of the second metatarsal is palpated and a mark is made on the skin immediately behind this. Then the head of the fifth metatarsal is palpated and a mark is made on the skin immediately behind it. Then, using the wetted lead of an indelible pencil or wet ink on the nib of a pen, the marks at the heads of the second and fifth metatarsals are joined by a straight line. This is the line of the lateral four metatarsal heads. Then the mark at the base of the head of the first metatarsal is joined to that at the base of the second metatarsal by a curved line, the curve following the contour of the easily palpable head of the first metatarsal.

While the marked lines are still wet, the patient is asked to stand down on a sheet of paper with his weight on the heel. He then carefully transfers his weight forward to the metatarsal heads *without* raising or moving the heel in any way. In this weight-bearing position, he remains standing while the designer outlines the whole foot accurately, even to the shapes of the toe tips. Great care must be taken to hold the pencil marking the outline in an upright position at all times. The sole of the foot bevels in before making contact with the paper, and if the marking pencil is slanted in or out, errors in width will be made.

Then the point of the pencil is placed just behind the head of the first metatarsal and is swept backward under the "arch" (waist) of the foot on the medial side, freely following the border of the sole of the foot as it comes in contact with the paper. This curved line gives the shoemaker the flat architectural "elevation" pattern. A further contour line is added later. Refer to Figures 9-4 and 9-5.

Next certain key measurements are made and recorded on the paper adjacent to the anatomical structures which are measured. A stiff shoemaker's tape is needed if the measurements are to be accurate. In Figure 11-1 these are designated as follows:

A. The height of the head of the first metatarsal head from the floor
B. The height of the fifth metatarsal head from the floor
C. The height of the navicula from the floor
D. The width across the foot at the metatarsal heads, best

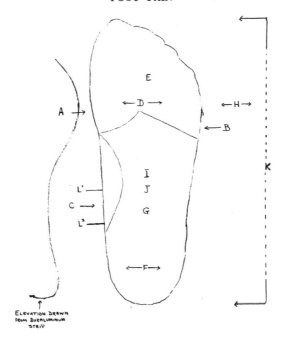

FIGURE 11-1.   The various measurements which have to be made
on a pattern to provide the bespoke shoemaker with adequate information from which he can alter a last in form with the foot.
The outline of the duraluminum impression is to the left. From this
the heel height is determined

measured with the shoe stick

E. The height of the highest interphalangeal joint of the toes

F. The width of the heel, best measured using the shoe stick

G. The measurement of the long heel (Fig. 11-2)

H. The circumference of the foot over the metatarsal heads
with the weight thrown forward on them

I. The circumference measurement of the seam standing
(Fig. 11-2)

J. The circumference of the instep standing (Fig. 11-2)

K. The length of the foot from heel to tip of the big toe

L. The designer lays his index and middle fingers together
across the dorsum of the foot, placed with the tarsonavicu-

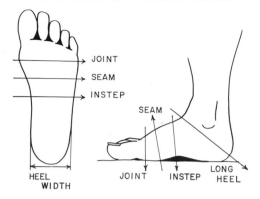

FIGURE 11-2.   The joint (H above), the seam (I above), the long
heel (G above), and the instep (J above) measurements.

lar joint between them, and marks the width of his two
fingers by lines on the medial aspect of the pattern

The patient then lifts his foot straight up off the paper onto
which the metatarsal head line has transferred, and further measurements are made of the foot without weight bearing.

M. The circumference of the foot over the metatarsal heads
N. The circumference measurement of the seam
O. The length of the long heel
P. The circumference of the instep
Q. The length of the foot from heel to tip of the big toe
R. Any vertical deformity of any toe

The vertical elevation is drawn from the shape of a duraluminum strip (Fig. 11-2), which is contoured to the inner border of
the foot from behind the heel to in front of the first metatarsal
head. This is also used to show the necessary heel height, which is
indicated by placing the front of the strip on the ground and raising the back of it until the heel part is horizontal to the floor (see
Figs. 9-2 and 9-3, pages 200–201).

Preparation of the Last. The shoemaker chooses a conventional last the length (size) of the foot using its standing measurement. He then has to alter the contour of the last by building it up with whittled pieces of leather — not forgetting to add a shaped toe piece ⅔ inch in length in front. In this way, when they are all in place, the various measurements of height and circumference of the last are identical with those taken from the feet, except that the width all around must be ¼ inch less overall, taking ⅛ inch from each side. Figures 11-3 and 11-4 illustrate normal lasts and how they are altered.

The Shoe Making. The foundation (which is the insole leather) having been mellowed, is blocked following exactly the plantar contours of the last. It is then trimmed and feathered to take the stitches which secure the welt to the upper. The upper

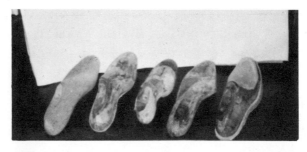

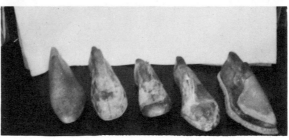

FIGURE 11-3. A normal last (*on the left of each picture*) and the various ways this may be altered from the measurements illustrated in Figure 11-1.

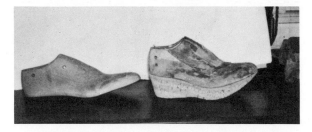

FIGURE 11-4. The rather complicated alteration of a last, together with the cork platform which is later incorporated in the shoe in place.

of the vamp and the quarter are roughed out (Figs. 11-5, 11-6, and 11-7 illustrate the various steps in shoe making). The platform insole is fashioned out of cork, just as though it were a support (see Chapter 9). Its undersurface is fitted to the foundation and stuck to it. The shank is affixed beneath the foundation in the long axis of the weight-bearing axis of the foot. The upper is softened and then molded carefully and snugly to the last. A toe stiffener and heel stiffener (counter) are added between the upper of the vamp and the quarter and their lining. The uppers are then trimmed before being sewn to the welt. At this point the shoe is ready for its first fitting. Seldom do changes

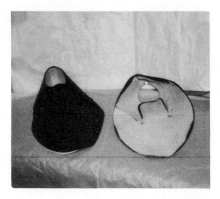

FIGURE 11-5. The upper of the vamp and quarter roughed out and lined before it is sewn to the welt of the foundation.

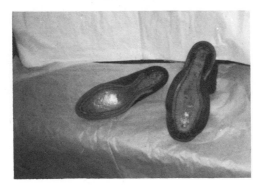

FIGURE 11-6.   The upper welted to the foundation, at which time
the shoe is ready for the fitting.

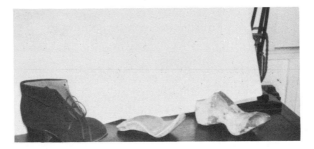

FIGURE 11-7.   The altered last on the right, the cork platform in
the center, and the finished shoe that is built around them on the
left.

need to be made except in the platform, which is readily filed away as necessary. It cannot be added to. Then when all is fitted, the sole and heel are attached and the shoe is complete.

The finer points of the art of construction cannot be put into words; they can be learned only by apprenticeship and experience.

12

Conclusion

The path of one who elects to care for patients with foot pain is strewn with rocks of frustration and paradox. The education gap in medical schools, and I dare to say in schools of podiatry, in problems of the musculoskeletal system compounds the difficulties.

Of patients who seek care for their foot pain, women are the bane of the doctor's existence. They are literally slaves to fashion. One might as well accept once and for all that one can neither adapt what women believe to be their "normal" shoes nor can bespoke shoes be styled to modern high fashion if they are to be made for comfort. Of women's shoes only those popularly called "wedgies," or oxfords with cuban heels, "Red Cross" nurse's shoes, or golf shoes without cleats lend themselves to adaptation. Even if it is possible to persuade a woman to give up fashion for comfort, it is usually necessary to compromise and even encourage the use of their fashionable shoes for party wear and other social occasions, providing they sit as much as possible on such occasions and even resort to kicking off their shoes under the dinner or bridge table.

One of the paradoxes is that women who most need foot care — the nurse, the waitress, the factory worker, and the poor housewife — can least afford it. And while mentioning cost I would make a plea to the professionals to survey their fee scale in the

237

light of the economic plight of the average patient suffering from foot pain. In my opinion it is outrageous, for instance, to charge anyone $125.00 for a pair of plastic supports which, even if they fit, cannot be changed from shoe to shoe. It is dishonest to undertake adaptation of high-fashion shoes for comfort.

There are stories which are apocryphal which highlight the problems of foot patients. One is about a poor young man who lived in the backwoods and who, on being called for induction into the armed services, walked 120 miles to the induction center where he was examined and rejected because of flatfeet. He then walked 120 miles back home and continued with his normal living with his painless, very functional feet.

I was appalled when I worked for the Veterans Administration at the number of men drawing lifetime pensions for permanent partial disability because of flatfeet or "foot problems." In these days of government spending cuts, I venture to say that a definite percentage of the pension budget deficit could be curtailed if this practice were to be eliminated at its source.

And, while talking of government problems, it seems to me that there is excellent opportunity for the poverty programs to train young men to be bespoke shoemakers. This is a highly skilled artistic trade — hard work certainly — and I suspect that the country could find full employment for at least a thousand of them. If the number of podiatrists employed by government installations such as Fort Bragg, which employs ten, can be used as an indication of the enormity of foot-care problems, then I suspect that every large army installation could find employment for at least two, every large Veterans Administration Hospital could absorb two, and every large medical center could absorb three or four. As a result of cunningly contrived Viet Cong booby traps, the Veterans Administration Hospitals are going to have to undertake lifetime treatment of disabled and partially destroyed feet. Only proper shoes can really help veterans disabled from such causes. Even if every city could not support one bespoke shoemaker, every state at least could support five or six even if they had to be employed as part of each State's Bureau of Vocational Rehabilitation, with a centralized shop, and be made available on an itinerant basis throughout the state.

There is a story of a Doctor Locke in Canada who used to sit in his "clinic" on a swivel stool in the center of a circle of patients with foot pain. Their shoes and socks were off. He would swivel around to each person in turn and manipulate their feet at fifty cents a time, giving probably not more than five minutes to each, and he is said to have made a fortune.

In my postgraduate classes held to teach manipulative examination and therapy, when we come to the feet we work on only one foot of each student. Invariably the students ask for the other foot to be mobilized afterward, as the worked-on foot is so comfortable. This prompts one to say again that if no one did anything more for people with painful feet (in the absence of gross disease) than mobilize all the joints of their feet, the incidence of foot pain would be decimated. Of course, this would have to be repeated at regular intervals if only mobilizing techniques were used and the skin, fascia, muscles, ligaments, bursae, and shoes were ignored.

It will always be difficult to persuade patients and insurance carriers that well-planned and well-carried-out physical therapy programs following personal injury are the most economical way of getting an individual back to independence and productivity. It is equally hard to persuade doctors and insurance carriers that good physical therapy cannot be carried out in doctors' offices by using this or that machine turned on and off by an office nurse or other aide. The prerequisite to good physical therapy is a well-trained Registered Physical Therapist. Unfortunately, even the executives of the American Physical Therapy Association are hard to convince of the immediate need for thousands more trained, working therapists to take care of the public's needs today. The expansion of the profession of physical therapy must be associated with an ongoing educational program for physicians in the care of musculoskeletal problems and the proper use of physical therapy in their treatment. But more physical therapy schools, and more physical therapists, are the prime need, and recognition of their professional status academically and economically is vital in order to attract students to this profession.

This book aims to demonstrate the methods of treatment exclusive of surgery which are available to the sufferer from foot pain at the hands of physicians and therapists. Foot pain is not a necessary evil, nor is surgery an inevitable choice of treatment. Education in this field of medicine is a crying need.

Bibliographic References

Billig Clinic. Symposium on foot problems confronted in industry, schools, the home and sports. *Int. Rec. Med.* 170:403–465, 1957.

Bowen, W. P. *Applied Anatomy and Kinesiology; The Mechanism of Muscular Movement* (7th ed.). (Revised by H. A. Stone.) Philadelphia: Lea & Febiger, 1953.

Brody, I. A., and Wilkins, R. H. Charcot-Marie-Tooth disease. *Arch. Neurol.* (Chicago) 17:552–557, 1967.

Burt, H. A. Effects of faulty posture. *Proc. Roy. Soc. Med.* 63:187–194, 1950.

Carlin, E. J. Functional osteology of the foot. *Phys. Ther. Rev.* 35:715–719, 1955.

Carlin, E. J. Special review — human gait. *Amer. J. Phys. Med.* 42:181–184, 1963.

Cherup, N., Urben, J., and Bender, L. F. The treatment of plantar warts with ultrasound. *Arch. Phys. Med.* 44:602–604, 1963.

Cholmeley, J. A. Hallux valgus in adolescents. *Proc. Roy. Soc. Med.* 51:903–906, 1958.

Cobey, M. C. The care and correction of congenital flatfoot. *Southern Med. J.* 51:586–590, 1958.

DeCoursey, R. M. *The Human Organism.* New York: McGraw-Hill, 1955.

Deyerle, W. M. The foot and lower leg. *Virginia Med. Monthly* 89:590–594, 1962.

DuVries, H. L. *Surgery of the Foot* (2d ed.). St. Louis: Mosby, 1965.

DuVries, H. L. Five myths about your feet. *Today's Health* 45:49–51, 1967.

Fields, A. Foot and Leg Cramps (Exhibit), A.M.A. Annual Convention, New York, 1965.)

Gelabert, R.   Anatomy for the dancer — with exercises to improve technique and prevent injury. *American Dancer* Vol. 1, 1927.

Griffin, J. E., Echternach, J. L., Price, R. E., and Touchstone, J. C. Patients treated with ultrasonic driven hydrocortisone and with ultrasound alone. *Phys. Ther.* 47:594–601, 1967.

Griffin, J. E., and Touchstone, J. C.   Ultrasonic movement of corticosteroids in pig tissues. *Proc. Soc. Exp. Biol. Med.* 109:461–463, 1962.

Hauser, E. D. W.   Management of lesions of the subtalar joint. *Surg. Clin. N. Amer.* 25:136–160, 1945.

Interglia, S.   Foot Problems and Their Remedies. Los Angeles: Orthopedic Shoe Last Clinic, Veterans Administration Center.

Keliklan, H.   *Hallux Valgus.* Philadelphia: Saunders, 1965.

Kent, H.   Plantar wart treatment with ultrasound. *Arch. Phys. Med.* 40:15–18, 1959.

Kidner, F. C.   The prehallux (accessory scaphoid) in its relation to flat foot. *J. Bone Joint Surg. [Amer.]* 11:831–837, 1929.

Mann, R., and Inman, V. J.   Phasic activity of intrinsic muscles of the foot. *J. Bone Joint Surg. [Amer.]* 48:469–481, 1964.

Mennell, J. B.   Foot gear. *Proc. Roy. Soc. Med.* 33:105–110, 1939.

Mennell, J. B.   *Physical Treatment by Mobilization and Massage* (5th ed.). London: Churchill, 1945.

Mennell, J. McM.   *Back Pain: Diagnosis and Treatment Using Manipulative Techniques.* Boston: Little, Brown, 1960.

Mennell, J. McM.   *Joint Pain: Diagnosis and Treatment Using Manipulative Techniques.* Boston: Little, Brown, 1964.

Morehouse, L. E.   Influence of a flexible outsole on the dynamics of the walking gait. *Int. Rec. Med.* 170:452–457, 1957.

Morton, D. J.   *The Human Foot, Its Evolution, Physiology and Functional Disorders.* New York: Columbia University Press, 1935.

Morton, T. G.   Peculiar and painful affection of the fourth metatarsophalangeal articulation. *Amer. J. Med. Sci.* 71:37–45, 1876.

Moseley, H. F.   Static disorders of the ankle and foot. *Ciba Clin. Symp.* 9:83–110, 1957.

Moseley, H. F.   Traumatic disorders of the ankle and foot. *Ciba Clin. Symp.* 17:3–30, 1965.

Munson, E. L.   *The Soldier's Foot and the Military Shoe.* Menasha, Wisconsin: Banta, 1917.

O'Brien, R. M.   Morton's toe. *Missouri Med.* 55:581–589, 1958.

Parscoe, J. Status report on those non-M.D. doctors. *Med. Econ.* January, 1961.

Peterson, L. T. My feet are killing me. *Med. Ann. D.C.* 34:118–121, 1965.

Pfizer Laboratories. My feet are killing me. *Spectrum* 14:54–55, 1966.

Pfizer Laboratories. Flatfoot — a common and preventable deformity of civilized man. *Spectrum* 9:66–68, 1961.

Podiatry and the Nation's Health. Washington, D.C.: American Podiatry Association.

Purves-Stewart, J., and Worster-Drought, C. *The Diagnosis of Nervous Diseases* (10th ed.). London: Arnold, 1952.

Quimby, H. R. *Pacemakers of Progress*. Chicago: Hide & Leather Publishing Co., 1946.

Root, L. Getting the most out of your feet. *Today's Health* 39:50–68, 1961.

Shands, A. R. Congenital defects of the skeleton. *Virginia Med. Monthly* 90:407–412, 1963.

Spalteholz, W. *Hand Atlas of Human Anatomy* (7th ed.). (Translated by Lewellys F. Barker.) Philadelphia: Lippincott, 1943.

Stein, H. C. The preservation of the function of the foot. *Clin. Orthop.* 4:123–151, 1954.

Travell, J., Baker, S., Hirsch, B., and Rinzler, S. H. Myofascial component of intermittent claudication. *Fed. Proc.* 11:164, 1952.

Veterans Administration, Department of Medicine and Surgery. Shoe modifications in lower-extremity orthotics. *Bull. Prosthetic Res.* Vol. 10, 1964.

Williams, M., and Worthingham, C. *Therapeutic Exercise in Body Alignment and Function*. Stanford, Calif.: Stanford University Press, 1953.

Winsor, T. *Peripheral Vascular Diseases*. Springfield, Ill.: Thomas, 1959.

Wright, D. G., and Rennels, D. C. A study of the elastic properties of plantar fascia. *J. Bone Joint Surg.* [*Amer.*] 48:482–492, 1964.

Index